Introduction to statistics for nurses

Visit the *Introduction to Statistics for Nurses* Companion Website at **www.pearsoned.co.uk/maltby** to find valuable **student** learning material including:

- Datasets from all four branches of Nursing that enable you to practise the exercises in the book
- Suggested solutions to all exercises in the book

We work with leading authors to develop the
strongest educational materials in nursing,
bringing cutting-edge thinking and best learning
practice to a global market

Under a range of well-known imprints we craft
high-quality print and electronic publications
which help readers to understand and apply
their content, whether studying or at work

To find out more about the complete range of our
publishing, please visit us on the World Wide Web at:
www.pearsoned.co.uk

Introduction to statistics for
nurses

John Maltby
School of Psychology, University of Leicester

Liz Day
School of Social Science and Law, Sheffield Hallam University

Glenn Williams
Psychology Division, School of Social Sciences, Nottingham Trent University

PEARSON
Education

Harlow, England • London • New York • Boston • San Francisco • Toronto
Sydney • Tokyo • Singapore • Hong Kong • Seoul • Taipei • New Delhi
Cape Town • Madrid • Mexico City • Amsterdam • Munich • Paris • Milan

Pearson Education Limited

Edinburgh Gate
Harlow
Essex CM20 2JE
England

and Associated Companies throughout the world

Visit us on the World Wide Web at:
www.pearsoned.co.uk

First published 2007

ISBN: 978-0-13-196753-3

British Library Cataloguing-in-Publication Data
A catalogue record for this book is available from the British Library

Library of Congress Cataloging-in-Publication Data
A catalog record for this book is available from the Library of Congress

10 9 8 7 6 5 4 3 2 1
11 10 09 08 07 06

Typeset in 9/13pt Interstate by 35
Printed by Ashford Colour Press Ltd., Gosport
The publisher's policy is to use paper manufactured from sustainable forests.

Contents

Chapter 3 Descriptive statistics: the Florence Nightingale way

Chapter 7   Correlational statistics   140

Chapter 8   Comparing average scores: statistics for all sorts of groups and occasions   169

Chapter 9 Critical appraisal of analysis and reporting of inferential statistics   216

Supporting resources

Visit **www.pearsoned.co.uk/maltby** to find valuable online resources

Companion Website for students

- Datasets from all four branches of Nursing that enable you to practise the exercises in the book
- Suggested solutions to all exercises in the book

For more information please contact your local Pearson Education sales representative or visit **www.pearsoned.co.uk/maltby**

List of figures

Preface

Introduction

We all constantly use statistics. Sometimes statistics are used to describe the different numbers in our lives. We know how much of our income we spend on different things, for example approximately how much on rent/mortgage payments, food and clothes. You would also be able to estimate what percentage of your income you spend on these things, and if not, you could still estimate that you spend a greater percentage of your income each month on your rent/mortgage than on clothes. We know roughly how much a week we spend. We know the average house prices on the street where we live. We could also find out from looking at the house prices which house in our neighbourhood is the most expensive and which is the cheapest.

Statistics in nursing are very similar. Nurses need to know about which sorts of patient have suffered the most side effects from a certain drug and which patients have had the fewest side effects. Nurses have to know what percentage of patients with a leg ulcer recover the quickest with a certain brand of dressing so that they can implement practice that is evidence based. Nurses should know about the likelihood that patients with a specific cancer will survive following early treatment by using facts and figures of survival rates. In the nursing profession, many of the things that affect a nurse's work have been guided by the use of statistics. For example, the use of a system of triage when assessing and admitting patients into accident and emergency departments will have been directed by statistical analysis of the amount of time staff can spend with patients and can feasibly provide an optimal level of care to them.

For many in the nursing profession, there is an increasing requirement to be statistically literate. Present-day pre-registration nursing students need statistical skills to become registered nurses. Even today's qualified nurses need to be able to understand and interpret a wide range of statistical tests to enable them to maintain satisfactory levels of continuing professional development and implement evidence-based practice. This book has been written with several audiences in mind, including:

- pre-registration nursing students on diploma in nursing courses who need to find out more about statistics and research methods, especially how to critique a study using quantitative methods (that is to say, the analysis of statistical information);
- undergraduate nursing students on a degree programme who are required to complete an empirical project to produce a dissertation;

● qualified nurses attending post-registration programmes that have modules dealing with research methods, statistics or the production of a dissertation.

Statistics can be an extremely useful tool. However, getting sufficient expertise in statistics can feel as if you are taking many steps on a long journey. We are keen to give you early success in applying statistics so that you can maintain your momentum and confidence in learning about this tool. This book is designed not only to help you experience early success by giving you working knowledge of a statistical package (SPSS for Windows), but also to enable you to gain the transferable skills for developing an understanding of statistics and how they are used in nursing research.

This book is designed for nurses who need to develop their knowledge and skills around statistics, but, more importantly, it aims to build your confidence through positive experience. We accept that many nurses find it difficult to use statistics or critique a study that has involved the use of statistics or are confused by the statistical jargon that is often used. This book is suitable for both qualified and unqualified nurses and will demystify many of these aspects. We seek to equip you with the skills to apply statistical techniques to analyse the evidence base for your nursing practice with the use of 'real-world' examples from nursing practice and research. We aim to offer you an accessible statistics book that does not assume prior statistical knowledge. We will be employing modern techniques of teaching and learning with the use of datasets and SPSS for Windows – one of the most widely used statistical software packages available on the market for nurses.

Most importantly, we have kept the book simple. We do not blind you with science or overload you with numbers; rather, we provide the simplest explanation of any concept so that you can learn statistics with confidence and ease.

Features

The book uses a variety of pedagogical features to help you in your study:

● Clear chapter objectives are presented in the form of **Key themes** and **Learning outcomes**, so you know the general areas that are addressed in each chapter and can check that you have covered all the major areas in the chapter.

● Each chapter opens with a **Case scenario.** These scenarios are labelled 'Imagine . . .' and give examples of where the use of statistics is relevant to you as a nurse. You are prompted to imagine that you are in a range of situations related to carrying out the job of the nurse. Some of these scenarios may even be ones that you have experienced. Each of these case scenarios is linked to topics covered in the chapter.

● From Chapter 3 onwards you will work through examples on SPSS using **four specially prepared datasets** which contain information specifically related to the four branches of nursing: adult, mental health, learning disability, and child. A number of research scenarios are used for tests that facilitate learning and develop transferable skills.

- **Self-assessment exercises** are provided at the end of most chapters so that you can check your own learning using the four datasets. There are also exercises within the text to allow you to check your progress towards understanding statistics in a research context. Answers or suggested answers to these exercises are available on the website accompanying this book at **www.pearsoned.co.uk/maltby**.

- Brief diversions are presented in boxes entitled **Point to consider**. These give additional information that expands upon, but is not essential to, each chapter's narrative.

- There are also **Task** and **Study** boxes which will allow you to test yourself on some of the material covered in the chapter.

- Key terms are highlighted in the text and collected together in a **glossary** at the end of the book.

Summary

The book aims to bring you success in using statistics by presenting a software package that is simple to use and by book chapters that can be completed in sessions of 1 to 2 hours. We hope you use the different methods we have tried to employ to support and facilitate your learning. By using this book, we are confident that you will be able to develop the knowledge and skills necessary to use statistics with confidence throughout your nursing career.

Acknowledgements

A big thank you to Kate for her guidance.

JM would also like to acknowledge the University of Leicester in granting him study leave to support the writing of this book.

Publisher's acknowledgements

Figures

Panels/screen shots showing SPSS software reproduced with permission from SPSS Inc.; Figures 10.3 and 10.4: Confidence Interval Calculator and Sample Size Calculator, reproduced with permission from Creative Research System.

Text

Box 2.2: Meikle, James (2000) 'Scientists warn of 30% rise in human BSE: What's wrong with our food?', *The Guardian*, 18 July 2000. © Guardian Newspapers Limited 2000, reproduced with permission; Box 2.3: Scott, Kirsty (2000) 'Miners' long hours blamed as lung disease returns', *The Guardian*, 18 July 2000. © Guardian Newspapers Limited, 2000, reproduced with permission; Box 2.6: Adrian O'Dowd (2006) 'The bigger picture: stress', *Nursing Times*, September 2006. Reproduced with permission; Box 9.2: Case 1 - Excerpts from W. Spence and W. El-Ansari (2004) 'Portfolio assessment: practice teachers' early experience', *Nurse Education Today*, 24: 388-401. Reproduced with permission from Elsevier Science.

In some instances we have been unable to trace the owners of copyright material, and we would appreciate any information that would enable us to do so.

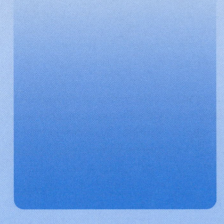

Chapter 1

An introduction to statistics

Key themes

✔ Introduction to statistics

✔ Why we use statistics

✔ What statistics are used for

✔ Thinking about statistics in their proper context

Learning outcomes

By the end of this chapter you will be able to:

✔ Understand statistics as a process for answering questions

✔ Understand that it is best to view statistics as a jigsaw, being made up of a number of parts forming an overall picture

Introduction

Imagine . . . You are a student nurse working in a cardiac care ward. During your first week, your mentor (a qualified nurse who oversees your training on placement) tells you about the treatments used on the ward. Your mentor mentions a treatment called statins and prompts you to find out about it. You are asked to do some reading about the evidence for, and against, statins as a treatment for patients after a heart attack. While reading the literature, you come across various results with lots of strange-looking symbols such as $p < 0.05$ and χ^2. This probably seems like a completely different world with the use of specialist statistical language and a wide array of numbers. You want to show your mentor that you can understand these studies but are unsure about what all these numbers and symbols mean. Maybe you'd like to do a research project of your own and analyse information about the use of statins on the ward compared with other types of treatment. How do you go about it? To test this type of question and many other research questions that affect your nursing career, you will need to use statistics.

At this stage it is likely that you feel you know nothing or very little about statistics. However, you've been using statistics all your life. We all constantly use statistics. Sometimes statistics are used to describe the different numbers in our lives. We know how much of our income we spend on different things, for example approximately how much on rent/mortgage payments, how much on food, how much on clothes. You would also be able to estimate what percentage you spend on these things, and if not, you could say that you spent a greater percentage of your income per month on your rent/mortgage than on clothes. We know roughly how much a week we spend (or can afford). We know the average house prices on the street where we live.

Some statistics are also used for looking at relationships between things. You also use these types of statistics all the time. You know, for example, that if you decorate a house you will probably raise its value (and if you neglect it, the house will decline in value). This shows a relationship between upkeep of your house and house prices. Similarly, you will have at some time read about differences in average income between men and women. Such statements are also based on a use of statistics.

These are everyday examples. In your profession as a nurse, you will be presented with statistics every day: mortality rates, average life expectancy, percentage recovery rate, average remission time, findings of which drugs work best with which illnesses, and relationships between level of care and remission rates for particular illnesses. Most of your job, the treatment strategies, the policies that surround your job and all the facts described above are derived from the use of statistics.

In the first few paragraphs we have subtly introduced you to all the aspects of statistics that will be required for the learning of statistics. That is, there is no statistical concept that we will introduce you to in this book that you haven't come across already in another context in your everyday or working life. To put it plainly, you already know a lot about some of the ideas that underlie statistics, because you come across them in all aspects of your life – you just don't know you know it yet.

In this first chapter we're going to tell you exactly what is going to happen in this book, as one of the problems with learning statistics is that beginners often don't have an overall picture of what they need to learn. This may lead to confusion: often concepts are learnt in isolation, without reference to the big picture. Liken this situation to knowing what happened at the end of a film. When you watch the film for a second time, you are able to appreciate plot developments and the significance of particular pieces of dialogue, and you notice events that seemed unimportant the first time but on a second viewing seem important. As you are unlikely to read this book again and again, we need to give the overview now.

There are two stages to this:

1   placing statistics within their proper context;
2   slotting together the different pieces of the statistics jigsaw to gain an overall picture.

Placing statistics and SPSS within their proper context

It is important that you understand why and what statistics are. Statistics are not a strange mystical force; rather, as we have already shown, they are something that you use every day in your life. However, in terms of nursing, let us see why statistics are important, and what statistics actually are.

Why do we use statistics?

Statistics constitute one part of a process (see Figure 1.1). At the beginning of any work using statistics, there is always an idea that the researcher expresses in the form of a question. The researcher will then collect some data designed to answer the question. Statistics are one tool that allows the researcher to provide answers to the research question; that is, statistics are one way to analyse data collected by a researcher. Therefore, it is important to view the use of statistics not as an isolated skill or something that exists separately from other things, but rather as a way of answering a question.

Let us illustrate. A new drug is on the market available for use with patients with heart complaints and you are asked to administer this drug. As a person who gives this drug to patients you want to be reassured that proper testing has been done to show that the drug works. You want to be confident in the use of that drug so that it doesn't produce dangerous side effects. As a result, you will seek out information in the British National Formulary or be given information about the drug to address your concerns.

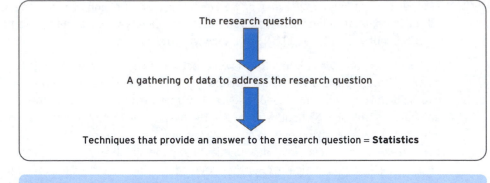

Figure 1.1 *Statistics are part of the research process*

Much of the information about the drug that will be used to address your concerns will be in the form of statistical data. Statistical data show you that patients administered the new drug have become healthier; they also show that there is a low risk of side effects when using that drug. In nursing there are many types of research question. Questions to do with clinical care (what is the relationship between treatment strategies and remission rates?), policy-based questions (does a new patient charter actually lead to improvement in care?), and professional questions (what aspects of the job attract nurses to the profession?).

So, why use statistics in nursing? Because statistics answer the questions that arise in your job.

What are statistics?

What actually are statistics? Statistics come in many forms, but they are basically one thing. They are a quantitative method of working out an answer to your question. By being quantitative, there are numbers or quantities that are used to show you the answers to your questions.

Remember when you were at school you were set a maths problem to which you had to find an answer. You would have a set of numbers, and you would have to carry out some procedure or apply some formula to those numbers to find the answer. That is the use of statistics. Statistics deal with numbers (or data) and help you make sense of them. They are no harder than the thinking you apply when you see a set of numbers such as

2, 4, 8, 16, 32, 64, 128, 256, 512.

Now look at these numbers for a second. You may have worked out two things about these numbers: that they are even numbers and that they double each time. Consider now this next set of numbers, and answer this question: which is the odd number out?

2, 4, 8, 16, 32, 17, 64, 128, 256, 512.

You would, particularly if you were using the rules above, have chosen 17. It is an odd number, and it doesn't fit into the pattern of each number doubling.

And that is the key to statistics. Statistics are no more than the operation of rules you apply to make sense of a set of numbers. The statistics that you will learn in this book are slightly more complicated than the rules of 'odd and even' and 'doubling', but they use the same basic idea of applying rules to understanding numbers.

There are techniques to help you apply these operations and rules. The most important techniques you will come across in this book use SPSS for Windows. What is SPSS for Windows? It is a computer program and its full name is the Statistical Package for the Social Sciences. It is used in a variety of academic disciplines, including nursing. To me and you it is a very advanced calculator, and extremely useful. Remember how a calculator helps you do complicated sums that you can't do in your head? SPSS's main aim is to save you time when working with numbers, particularly when you have lots of calculations to do. It can perform complicated operations, and it doesn't make mistakes. We will introduce you to these different parts of the SPSS computer program as we work through the book.

In sum, what this section should have shown you is that it is important to view statistics as a tool for understanding numbers and answering your questions. It is there to aid you in your understanding of the numbers that surround you in your job. You should not let your feelings about maths or numbers lead you to feel that statistics are in charge of or central to the research process. You and the question you want answered are central to the process. Statistics are there to help you.

Overview of statistics: the jigsaw

We've told you what statistics are and that there are different types. But let us now give you an overview of the different aspects that you will encounter in this book. There are a number of different parts to statistics. Each of these parts is important in providing an overall view. Therefore, we think a knowledge of statistics is a little like a jigsaw puzzle (see Figure 1.2a). By putting all the different parts together you can effectively apply statistics (Figure 1.2b).

In this book we have used each chapter to address each piece of this jigsaw. The chapters represent all the outside blocks, starting with variables in Chapter 2.

To place statistics in context, it is worthwhile summarising the main points of each chapter here. Don't worry if this seems overwhelming at this stage: we will address all these concepts in detail within each of the chapters. However, by surveying some of them now we can give you a real sense of the overall picture of statistics.

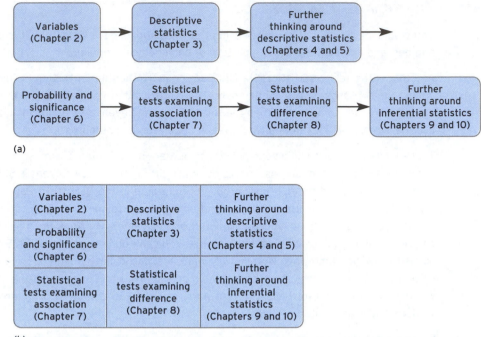

(a)

(b)

Figure 1.2 *(a) The separate parts of the statistical jigsaw. (b) How the separate parts of the statistical jigsaw come together*

Chapter 2: Variables

Chapter 2 is designed to teach you some core ideas that underlie statistics. By the end of this chapter you will be able to:

● outline what variables are and how they are evident in many aspects of investigation;

● describe how variables are viewed by investigators;

● demonstrate the form variables take in SPSS for Windows by way of creating a datafile;

● use SPSS for Windows to create and save a datafile of variables.

Chapter 3: Descriptive statistics

Chapter 3 is designed to teach you ways of describing data. By the end of this chapter you will be able to:

● demonstrate knowledge of frequency counts, averages, a measure of dispersion, bar charts and histograms, and how to obtain these statistics on SPSS for Windows;

- perform, in SPSS for Windows, techniques in statistics that allow you to alter the structure of your data: the Recode and Compute commands.

Chapter 4: Effective data cleaning and management

Chapter 4 is designed to teach you ways of managing statistical data. By the end of this chapter you will be able to:

- examine the concept of validity and explain why it is important in nursing research;
- make the data collected more valid by using proper techniques of data cleaning and management;
- use descriptive statistics to look for errors in data entry or coding.

Chapter 5: Critical appraisal of analysis and reporting of descriptive statistics

Chapter 5 is designed to teach you ways of thinking further about descriptive statistics. By the end of this chapter you will be able to:

- explain the importance of critical appraisal as a process for evaluating strengths and limitations of a study;
- outline a critical appraisal framework for evaluating the use of descriptive statistics in a study;
- apply your critical appraisal skills by using the critical appraisal framework to evaluate a case study article.

Chapter 6: An introduction to inferential statistics

Chapter 6 is designed to introduce you to a series of statistical tests called inferential statistics. By the end of this chapter you will be able to:

- outline what is meant by terms such as distribution, probability and statistical significance testing;
- outline the importance of probability values in determining statistical significance;
- outline the decision-making process about what informs the use of parametric and non-parametric statistical tests;
- determine a statistically significant result;
- carry out your first inferential statistical test using SPSS for Windows, the chi-square test.

Chapter 7: Correlational statistics

Chapter 7 is designed to teach you about two types of inferential statistical tests known as correlation statistics. By the end of this chapter you will learn the rationale for, the procedure for and the interpretation in SPSS for Windows of two inferential statistical tests:

- Pearson product-moment correlation;
- Spearman's rho correlation.

Chapter 8: Comparing average scores

Chapter 8 is designed to teach you about four types of inferential statistical test that are concerned with examining differences. By the end of this chapter you will learn the rationale for, the procedure for and the interpretation in SPSS for Windows of the following four inferential statistical tests:

- independent-samples *t*-test;
- paired-samples *t*-test;
- Wilcoxon sign-ranks test;
- Mann–Whitney *U* test.

Chapter 9: Critical appraisal of analysis and reporting of inferential statistics

Chapter 9 is designed to help you understand the use of inferential statistics in nursing research papers and the nursing literature. The chapter contains sections which will ask you to interpret examples from the literature. By the end of this chapter you will be able to:

- use critical appraisal to evaluate the reporting of inferential statistics;
- apply a critical appraisal framework to evaluate research and research articles – in this case, how well a fictitious article (based on the adult branch dataset) has adhered to the issues raised in the critical appraisal framework.

Chapter 10: Advanced thinking with probability and significance

Chapter 10 is designed to teach you about thinking further around inferential statistical tests. Therefore, at the end of this chapter you should be able to outline ideas of:

- statistical and clinical significance, and how these relate to effect size and percentage improvement;
- hypothesis testing and confidence intervals, and how these two concepts are used in the literature to provide context to statistical findings.

Summary

Now you know about the main areas and issues that underlie statistics. In terms of what you need to have learnt from this chapter, there are two important things to remember:

✔ Statistics are part of a process – a process for answering a question.

✔ Statistics are about knowledge of the use of numbers; they come together as a whole. Therefore, it is best to view statistics as a jigsaw, being made up of a number of parts forming an overall picture.

In the next chapter we introduce you to the first piece of the statistics jigsaw: variables.

Chapter 2

Variables

Key themes

✔ Variables

✔ Types of variable

✔ Data entry in SPSS for Windows

Learning outcomes

By the end of this chapter you will be able to:

✔ Outline what variables are and how they are evident in many aspects of investigation

✔ Describe how variables are viewed by researchers

✔ Demonstrate the form variables take in SPSS for Windows by way of creating a datafile

✔ Use SPSS for Windows to create and save a datafile of variables

Introduction

How do you view the world? Do you view it as made up of good and evil, of right wing political thought or left wing political thought, or of those who are rich and those who are poor? Or do you view the world in terms of your profession, those who care for others, and those who are cared for? Or those who are well or those who are ill? In this chapter we are going to introduce you to another way of viewing the world . . . that is, by seeing the world as made up of variables.

Imagine . . . That you are a leg ulcer specialist nurse and are trying to decide on the most effective methods for dressing your patients' leg ulcers – do you use a short-stretch bandage or a medium-stretch one? How would you assess the effectiveness of the dressing? Through its (1) comfort, (2) ability to alleviate pain or (3) effect on how quickly the leg ulcer heals? All three ways of looking at the effectiveness of a type of dressing can be labelled 'variables' as they can vary for different groups of patients and depending on how severe the leg ulcer is (another variable). We will be identifying more variables in this chapter as the notion of having variables to analyse is the cornerstone of any statistics that you will be doing in your studies and your nursing career.

The idea of *variables* is central to statistics. In this chapter we are going not only to tell you what variables are but also to get you working with them. You use variables every day in your life (the time you get up in the morning, the amount of money you spend on different things during the day), and the notion that many things are variables in your life is a key aspect of statistics. What we will show you in this chapter is how variables can be understood and defined in our lives, which then will give you a powerful basis for understanding some of our later points about statistics.

In this chapter you will explore:

- what variables are, and how they are evident in many aspects of investigation;
- how variables are viewed by researchers;
- the form that variables take in SPSS for Windows by way of creating a datafile;
- how to use SPSS for Windows to create and save a datafile of variables.

Energiser

Before we start, let us do a little exercise. This task is designed to get you thinking about variables. In your nursing practice, you will need to handle different ways of measuring things, ranging from assessing a patient's health needs to seeing how well a treatment has worked. In Box 2.1, write down in the space provided the things that you may need to measure in your everyday practice. Also, write down in the second column how you measure these things. Three examples have been provided to give you some ideas.

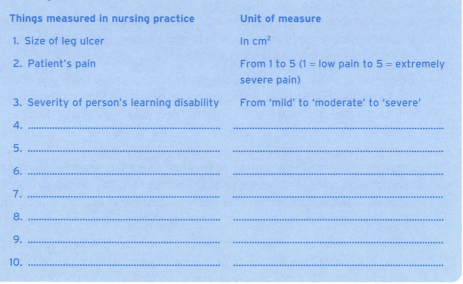

Box 2.1 Task

Energiser table

Things measured in nursing practice	Unit of measure
1. Size of leg ulcer	In cm²
2. Patient's pain	From 1 to 5 (1 = low pain to 5 = extremely severe pain)
3. Severity of person's learning disability	From 'mild' to 'moderate' to 'severe'
4.	....
5.	....
6.	....
7.	....
8.	....
9.	....
10.	....

Variables

Variables are quite simply things that vary. We are surrounded by variables. Examples of variables are: different types of events or objects, our feelings and attitudes, and other people's feeling and attitudes. Instances of these could be the different times that people get up in the morning, the different types of breakfast they might have (if any), the way that people feel about work, the number of hours they spend watching television at night, and the time they go to bed. These examples are slightly flippant, but valid. As researchers we tend to be interested in those variables related to our discipline. An economist would be interested in interest rates, unemployment figures, and levels of supply and demand. However, as nurses, you will be most interested in how well patients recover after becoming ill, the different types of illness they face, and the treatment options available to them.

Identifying variables

One important skill that researchers must have is to be able to identify accurately the variables which exist in an area of research. We are going to spend a little time looking at how to develop the skill of identifying variables.

Read the article by James Meikle in Box 2.2.

You will see that there are many variables in which government scientists are interested. At one level it may seem that scientists are interested only in the levels of vCJD, and in how many people have died of vCJD. However, there are other variables that can be identified within this article:

- the year people have died in (to consider trends in the disease);
- changes in the frequency of vCJD, by looking at changes from one year to the next;
- the time period between which 'friends, relatives or doctors first noted the symptoms' and eventual death, which varies from 7 to 38 months;
- whether people have died of vCJD or another related disease;
- where the vCJD case occurred. Here there is an emphasis on Queniborough in Leicestershire.

We can see, therefore, that even within a fairly straightforward area of research, many variables emerge during the course of an investigation.

Box 2.2 Task

Scientists warn of 30% rise in human BSE

Government scientists yesterday warned of a sharply accelerating trend in the incidence of human BSE after studying the pattern of the disease so far.

They said the number of reported cases may in fact be rising at between 20% and 30% a year despite the apparently varied annual death rates over the past five years.

The prediction came as it was revealed that the death toll from the incurable condition officially known as vCJD had risen by a further two in the past fortnight to a total of 69, and 14 so far this year.

The scientists said that there was now a 'statistically significant rising trend' in the number of victims since the first casualties first displayed signs of the disease in 1994, although it was still too early to forecast the ultimate number of deaths caused by vCJD.

This year's toll is already equal to that for the whole of last year when the number dropped. A further seven people still alive are thought to be suffering from the condition. The scientists have come to their conclusion about the progress of the disease after analyses of monthly figures, including studying the dates at which friends, relatives or doctors first noted symptoms.

The period between this and eventual death has varied between seven and 38 months, with an average of 14 months, although the incubation period before symptoms become evident is believed to be several years longer.

Stephen Churchill was the first known death from the disease in May 1995, although it was not formally identified or officially linked to the eating of beef in the late 1980s until March 1996. Three people died in 1995, 10 in 1996, 10 in 1997, 18 in 1998 and 14 last year.

Members of the government's spongiform encephalopathy advisory committee took the unusual step of publishing the figure immediately after their meeting in London yesterday because of the recent interest in a cluster of five cases around Queniborough in Leicestershire.

These included three victims dying within a few of months in 1998, a fourth who died in May and another patient, still alive, who is thought to be suffering from the same disease.

The scientists said this was 'unlikely to have occurred by chance but this cannot be completely ruled out' and they would be closely informed about local investigations. The Department of Health last night said it could not elaborate on the significance of the new analysis until ministers and officials had considered the scientists' new advice.

The figures came amid reports that sheep imported by the US from Europe were showing signs of a disease, which could be linked to BSE in cattle. Government scientists are to hold talks with their US counterparts after the US agriculture department ordered the destruction of three flocks of sheep, which were in quarantine in the state of Vermont.

Source: James Meikle, 'Scientists warn of 30% rise in human BSE: What's wrong with our food?', The Guardian, 18 July 2000. © The Guardian Newspapers Limited, 2000, reproduced with permission.

A useful thinking skill that you can develop is to be able to identify what possible variables are contained within a research area. Read the next article by Kirsty Scott, which appeared in the same issue of *The Guardian* (Box 2.3). Try to identify, and list in the box, as many variables as you can see emerging from this report. You should be able to name several.

Box 2.3 Task

Miners' long hours blamed as lung disease returns

Miners at a Scottish colliery are suffering from a serious lung disease that health experts thought had been virtually eradicated.

Routine tests have found that nine miners at the Longannet colliery in Fife have developed pneumoconiosis, or black lung, which is caused by inhaling coal dust.

A further 11 have abnormalities in the lungs, an early stage of the condition. The condition, which can lead to debilitating and sometimes fatal respiratory disease, was thought to have almost disappeared with the introduction of new safety and screening measures in the mid-1970s.

Last year a compensation scheme was agreed for miners affected by the disease after the biggest ever personal injury action in the UK. A health and safety executive report on the Longannet findings is expected to blame excessive working hours and a failure to use protective equipment properly.

Dan Mitchell, HSE chief inspector of mines, said it was unusual to have found such an outbreak. 'But certainly in recent years the number of workers in mines attending for x-ray has been falling,' he said. 'It's not as good as it used to be and we only know about the prevalence of disease from the people who are x-rayed.'

The re-emergence of the disease has also surprised medical authorities at the Scottish pulmonary vascular unit at the Western Infirmary in Glasgow. 'I am really quite surprised because we have known about this condition for years and screening measures have been in place for years,' said the unit head, Andrew Peacock. 'We know what causes it. We expect old cases from the past but new cases coming along now does surprise me.'

Under regulations introduced in 1975 miners are only supposed to work 7-hour shifts, but many work overtime. They are also expected to have lung x-rays every five years, but at Longannet only around 70% of men took part on the last occasion.

Representatives from the National Union of Mineworkers met HSE officials yesterday to discuss the situation. Peter Neilsen, vice-president of the NUM in Scotland, said: 'We thought that disease had disappeared. As a union we are concerned and it is our intention to take stock of the situation.'

The Scottish Coal Deep Mine Company, which runs Longannet, issued a statement saying that health of employees was of the utmost concern. More than 82,000 claims for compensation have been filed since the miners won their health case against the government and the nationalised coal industry. They claimed it had been known for decades that dust produced in the coal mining process could cause diseases like emphysema and chronic bronchitis and that not enough was done to protect them.

Now list as many variables as you can find in the above article.

....

....

....

....

....

● Identifying variables within academic titles and text

What is particularly interesting about the example in Box 2.3 is that the report begins to speculate about some of the causes of lung cancer. The researchers suggest that a number of different variables have contributed to lung disease. These include whether workers have worked excessive hours, the number of times they may have worked excessive hours, and whether protective equipment is worn.

Also, being able to identify how variables relate to other variables is central to any research. All researchers are interested in asking, and trying to answer, research questions about the relationships between variables. Some researchers will refer to research questions in different ways. Some researchers refer to hypotheses, aims or objectives, but basically these are terms used to answer a question about research. Therefore, a research question a nurse might ask is whether smoking (Variable 1: whether a person smokes) is a cause of heart disease (Variable 2: whether a person develops heart disease).

So far, we have used examples where researchers may be seeking to establish connections between variables. However, it is also worth noting that researchers are sometimes equally interested in not finding relationships between variables. For example, a research nurse would be interested in ensuring that a new drug does not have any major side effects.

Exercise: Identifying variables

Using the captions from the newspaper articles in Box 2.4, try to identify the variables and what possible links the journalists and researchers are trying to identify and establish.

Box 2.4 Task

Try identifying variables from these headlines from a variety of nursing publications

Adult branch nursing articles

'Cold comfort: the impact of poverty on older people's health', *Nursing Standard* (2004) 19(5): 1

'Pain-free heart attacks raise risk of death', *Nursing Times* (2004) 100(33): 6

....

....

Learning disability branch nursing articles

'The impact of nurse education on staff attributions in relation to challenging behaviour', *Learning Disability Practice* (2004) 7(5): 16

'Choice-making for people with a learning disability', *Learning Disability Practice* (1998) 1(3): 22

....

....

Mental health branch nursing articles

'Half of mental health service users back concept of compulsory home treatment', *Nursing Times* (2004) 100(41): 5

'The role of lithium clinics in the treatment of bipolar disorder', *Nursing Times* (2004) 100(27): 42

....

....

Child branch nursing articles

'Sedentary kids more likely to get ME', *Nursing Times* (2004) 100(41): 9

'How nurse intervention is tackling child obesity', *Nursing Times* (2004) 100(31): 26

....

....

Repeat the exercise with some academic journal titles (Box 2.5).

Box 2.5 Task

Try identifying variables from these journal article titles

'Symptoms of anxiety and depression among mothers of pre-school children: effect of chronic strain related to children and child care-taking' (Naerde *et al.*, 2000)

....

....

'Characteristics of severely mentally ill patients in and out of contact with community mental health services' (Barr, 2000)

....

....

'Gender and treatment differences in knowledge, health beliefs, and metabolic control in Mexican Americans with type B diabetes' (Brown *et al.*, 2000)

....

....

Distinctions *within* variables

Now that we know how to identify a variable, we need to understand that certain distinctions are made within variables. These distinctions are called levels of a variable, and are quite simply the different elements that exist within a variable. Therefore, all variables have a number of levels. Sex of a person has two levels: you are a man or a woman. Age has numerous levels ranging from birth to a probable maximum of 120 years old. We have seen levels in all the examples we have used so far. Take, for example, the variables we identified in the vCJD article:

- *The year people have died*. The levels here are the years 1992, 1993, 1994 and so on.
- *The time period between which 'friends, relatives or doctors first noted the symptoms' and eventual death, which varies from 7 to 38 months*. The levels here are in months.
- *Whether people have died from vCJD or a related disease*. The levels here could be twofold. The first version might contain only two levels, those being (1) whether the person had died of vCJD, or (2) whether the person had died not of vCJD but of a related disease. A second version might contain levels that describe each related disease, leading to many more levels.
- *Where the vCJD case occurred*. Here there is an emphasis on Queniborough in Leicestershire. The levels here are different places, for example Leicestershire, Nottinghamshire, Derbyshire.

Distinctions *between* types of variable

You now know you can make distinctions within variables. We now need to expand on these distinctions and understand that researchers then go on to make distinctions *between* different types of variable. The main reason for these distinctions is that they underpin the choices that need to be made when using a statistical test. There are two common sets of distinctions that researchers make between variables. These distinctions rely on how researchers view the levels that exist within a variable.

● Set 1: distinctions between nominal, ordinal, interval and ratio

In this set, the first type of variable is called **nominal** and this entails merely placing levels into separate categories. The levels of this variable type (a nominal variable) are viewed as distinct from one another. For example, the sex of a person has two levels: male and female. As sex is biologically determined, individuals fall into one category or the other. There are other nominal variables such as classification of dressings (for example, multi-layer versus short-stretch bandages) or variables taken from something like the ICD-10 classification system, which categorises medical conditions and treatments.

The next type of variable in this set is called **ordinal**, and this means that the levels of the variable can be placed into ranked ordered categories. However, the categories do not have a numerical value. A healthcare-related example is a pain rating score ranked from 0 to 3. One patient could have no pain (scored as 0), one could have mild pain (scored as 1), another could have moderate pain (scored as 2) and another patient could have extremely severe pain (scored as 3). We can see that although levels of pain go up with the scores given for each response, representing greater and greater pain, they do not represent equal differences between the categories that are suggested by the numbers. For example, there is a gap of 1 between mild pain (1) and moderate pain (2). But, is this equal to the gap of 1 between moderate pain (2) and severe pain (3)? Therefore, the numbers that are assigned are arbitrary but are designed to give some indication of levels of pain.

The next types of variable are **interval** and **ratio**. The levels for both these variables are numerical, meaning that they comprise numerical values. These numbers do not represent something else, in the way that the numbers used above for the ordinal variable do, for rating pain. However, there is a distinction between interval and ratio variables. Ratio data have an absolute zero, in other words they can have an absence of the variable, whereas interval data do not have an absolute zero. So, for example, the number of children in a family is a ratio variable because families can have no children.

Interval variables do not have an absolute zero. Common examples of interval variables are many concepts we use in everyday life, such as self-esteem. The measurement of self-esteem is not readily available to us (as opposed to simply counting the number of people in a family). Measurement of self-esteem in research will normally involve adding together the responses to a number of questions to produce a self-esteem scale. Consequently we refer to self-esteem in terms of low or high self-esteem, or relative terms, such as a person having higher, or lower, self-esteem than another person. Because of this type of measurement we can, at no point, establish that there is an absence of self-esteem (in other words that there is an absolute zero), so researchers treat many scales as interval data.

● Set 2: distinctions between categorical, discrete and continuous

The other set of distinctions comprises those that are made between **categorical**, **discrete** and **continuous** variables. Categorical data are the same as nominal data. Yet in this set of distinctions, researchers make an important distinction between discrete and continuous data. Here, both these variables are numerical. However, continuous variables allow for decimal points (for example 10.5678 cm^2 of the total pressure sore area), whereas discrete data do not allow for decimal points (you can't get 3.5 patients waiting on trolleys in the ward).

● Combining sets 1 and 2: categorical-type and continuous-type variables

As you can see from these two sets of distinctions between types of variables, there are different ways that researchers make distinctions between variables (and there are also a number of ways in which people merge these different sets of definitions and develop different understandings). Having different definitions can be terribly confusing for people starting out in statistics. This is sometimes particularly difficult, as teachers of statistics will adopt different definitions. If you are on a course you will probably, in time, come across different teachers who use different ways of defining variables.

To put it simply, one of the main sources of possible confusion is how teachers of statistics differ in the way they view the ordinal variable (set 1) and the discrete variable (set 2). There are two possible ways in which researchers perceive both types of variable. For many researchers, both ordinal and discrete variables are essentially ordered in a numerical way, and as such they believe that they should be viewed in the same way as continuous/interval/ratio variables.

However, for other researchers, ordinal and discrete variables represent separate, unique levels that do not represent numbers on a continuum. One example often cited, to support the latter point, is the distance represented *between* the levels of an ordinal variable. Unlike for numerical variables, in which the distance between levels is equal (the distance between 1 and 2, and 2 and 3, and 3 and 4, is the same, 1), for ordinal data, the distances between the levels are not the same (for example, in the example of the pain ratings above, the distances between severe, moderate and mild pain may not be of equal value).

However, there is a simple strategy (see Figure 2.1) with which to tackle this issue without confusion when beginning statistics (this is by no means foolproof but it provides a useful survival technique). This strategy relies on emphasising the similarities between

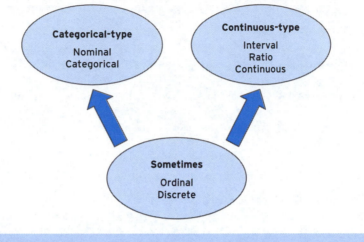

Figure 2.1 Simple strategy for remembering distinctions between variables

the two descriptions, rather than the differences. Within this strategy, variables can instead be treated as either

- categorical-type (distinct levels), or
- continuous-type (numerical ordered levels).

This means that, in the first instance, you should think of nominal/categorical variables as merely **categorical-type data** (variables that form separate categories). You should then think of ordinal/interval/ratio/discrete/continuous variables as merely **continuous-type data** (variables that form a series of numbers, that either rise or lower in value).

However, you must always remember that different researchers treat ordinal and discrete variables differently. Some researchers insist that these variables are categorical and some insist that they are continuous. As such, there is no right or wrong view. Rather, you just have to be aware that this distinction occurs. This distinction has some implications for choosing which statistical test to use; we will return to this issue in Chapter 6 when an overall guide to the process of choosing which statistical test to use will be presented. However, the employment of this strategy will allow you to navigate through the statistics contained in this book.

Identifying variables

Using the article 'The bigger picture: stress' (Box 2.6), identify the variables (and the possible levels within the variables). For the variables you identify, note whether the variable is categorical or continuous. If you are feeling confident you may even make further distinctions between types of variable (i.e. is the variable nominal/categorical, ordinal, interval, ratio, discrete, continuous?). Some possible answers are given on the book's website at **www.pearsoned.co.uk/maltby**.

Box 2.6 Task

The bigger picture: stress

Stress is a part of nursing, just as it is in many professions and workplaces. Nursing, however, is considered as one of the most stressful of occupations as it involves hard, intense work and deals with life and death situations.

The Health and Safety Executive (HSE) rates nursing as the second most stressful occupation, only beaten by teaching.

In simple terms, stress is a temporary imbalance in a person's emotional state and behaviour, usually happening when people are under more pressure than they can cope with. Most people believe that a little stress can be good to make them perform better, but if allowed to continue and get out of control, stress can lead to serious side-effects such as physical sickness and depression.

The impact of too much stress on nurses is important because the psychological and mental harm caused by stress can adversely affect how they deliver patient care, it can cause distress to the nurse themselves, and it can affect their health and attendance record.

Nationally, around 16% of all workers say their jobs are 'very' or 'extremely' stressful, according to a survey by the HSE of 3,800 people carried out in 2005.

In healthcare the levels seem to be higher and a Healthcare Commission survey of 217,000 NHS staff in 2004 found that 36% of people said they were suffering from work-related stress.

The cost of stress is significant and the HSE estimates that 6.5 million working days are lost in the UK every year because of stress. The problem of workplace stress is calculated to cost the UK economy £7 billion a year.

It is not only the life and death nature of what nurses do that can make the work stressful, but also excessive workload, reliance on agency staff, relationships between nurses and other professions and being unable to switch off when they go home.

A good employer should have policies on managing stress to help their employees, but not all do. Some trusts have confidential staff counselling services, for example, and some train managers in stress management policy so they can identify and reduce staff stress.

> Individuals can help to minimise stress themselves by taking regular exercise, eating a balanced diet, and getting plenty of sleep and relaxation. More assertive people will be better at coping with stress as they will say 'no' to things quicker and find it easier to ask for help and support.
>
> *Source:* Adrian O'Dowd (2006) 'The bigger picture : stress', *Nursing Times*, September 2006. Reproduced with permission.

Wider context of data-collecting research and SPSS for Windows

The next stage in this process is to begin to convert variables into usable data to answer a research question. This follows a process:

1   Collect the data.

2   Give the data some codes.

3   Enter these codes into a datasheet on SPSS for Windows.

● Collecting the data

To collect variable data you would usually ask questions of a number of people. This could be done in several ways. The most common in statistics would be via a questionnaire, experiment or one-to-one interview. The different ways in which you can collect data is a subject more for research methods than for statistics books. What we are concerned with here is how you begin the analysis of the data. However, in order to demonstrate this stage, we need to provide some data. We are going to use data that we have generated from four people, who answered the questionnaire shown in Figure 2.2.

● Coding the data

First, we must convert all the variables and their separate levels into numbers. This happens because all statistical packages tend to use number codes to deal with variables because they are mathematical machines. Researchers code all variables into

Please answer these questions by circling the appropriate response or filling in the gap

Question 1: Are you   Male   or   Female?

Question 2: What age are you? _____ years

Question 3: What bandage are you using for your leg ulcer?

        Medium-stretch   or   Short-Stretch

Question 4: How much pain is your leg ulcer giving you?

        None   Mild   Moderate   Severe

Figure 2.2 *The leg ulcer survey*

numbers regardless of whether the variables are numerical. This should not intimidate you. You simply decide what the number codes are for each variable. So, for our example, where we have asked respondents what sex they are, they indicate whether they are male or female. You would then, in preparing the data for coding, assign a code for each category. Usually this would be 1 for male and 2 for female (or vice versa). It is not worth coding the question about age into numbers, as each response is already a number. We would repeat this process for all the other variables. For the 'bandage' variable, we would assign 1 for medium-stretch and 2 for short-stretch bandaging. For the pain variable, it would be 1 for none, 2 for mild, 3 for moderate and 4 for severe.

● Entering data into a datasheet on SPSS for Windows: the principles

An important skill in this part of the analysis process is to be able to visualise the way in which data are laid out. To make this skill explicit, we are going to use an example on paper (the next section shows how to do this on SPSS for Windows).

Data are laid out in SPSS for Windows in a grid format (Figure 2.3). In this grid the columns represent different variables, and the rows will represent each person (respondent). What you aim to do then is to fill the grid with all the information you have gathered.

Let us use the data collected from the four people on their sex, age, bandage type and pain level.

- Respondent 1 was male, aged 29, used a medium-stretch bandage and was in mild pain.

- Respondent 2 was female, aged 32, used a short-stretch bandage and was in moderate pain.

	Sex	Age	Bandage	Ulcer pain
Respondent 1				
Respondent 2				
Respondent 3				
Respondent 4				

Figure 2.3 A data grid for the leg ulcer survey

- Respondent 3 was male, aged 25, used a medium-stretch bandage and was in moderate pain.
- Respondent 4 was male, aged 28, used a short-stretch bandage and was in severe pain.

Using the codes that we created in the previous subsection, we would assign the following code for each person:

- Respondent 1: Sex = 1, Age = 29, Bandage = 1, Ulcer pain = 2.
- Respondent 2: Sex = 2, Age = 32, Bandage = 2, Ulcer pain = 3.
- Respondent 3: Sex = 1, Age = 25, Bandage = 1, Ulcer pain = 3.
- Respondent 4: Sex = 1, Age = 28, Bandage = 2, Ulcer pain = 4.

These would then be transferred on to the grid, as in Figure 2.4, putting each number in the appropriate box, according to where it lies within the columns and row.

This is the essence of how data are entered and presented in SPSS for Windows. In the next section we show you how to do this in practice using the software. However, before we do this, try the following exercise.

	Sex	Age	Bandage	Ulcer pain
Respondent 1	1	29	1	2
Respondent 2	2	32	2	3
Respondent 3	1	25	1	3
Respondent 4	1	28	2	4

Figure 2.4 Completed data grid for the leg ulcer survey

	Sex	Age	Bandage	Ulcer pain
Respondent 1	2	29	2	4
Respondent 2	1	35	1	3
Respondent 3	2	38	2	3
Respondent 4	1	55	2	1

Figure 2.5 *Data grid for exercise: using a dataset*

Exercise: Using a dataset

Using the coding for sex, age, bandage and pain, answer the following questions for the dataset in Figure 2.5.

1 What is the type of bandage worn by respondent 2?

2 How many males are experiencing moderate or severe pain?

3 How many respondents are using the medium-stretch bandage?

Entering data on SPSS for Windows

When you start up SPSS for the first time, the first window that you see will be SPSS's data grid (Figure 2.6), which, in effect, is a spreadsheet (matrix of columns reading downwards and rows reading across). You use this sheet to enter your data in SPSS, and it is very similar to the layout of the grids we used in the previous section. In this section we will learn how to type data into SPSS.

Before typing in data we need to do two things: (1) collect the data to type in, and (2) prepare the SPSS file for data entry.

Collecting data

For this example we collected data from five respondents who answered the questionnaire shown in Figure 2.7. Their answers are shown in Figure 2.8.

We now have our data, so let us create a datafile in SPSS for Windows.

Preparing the SPSS datafile

Before typing in the data, it is considered good practice to prepare the variables in the dataset. This comprises four stages:

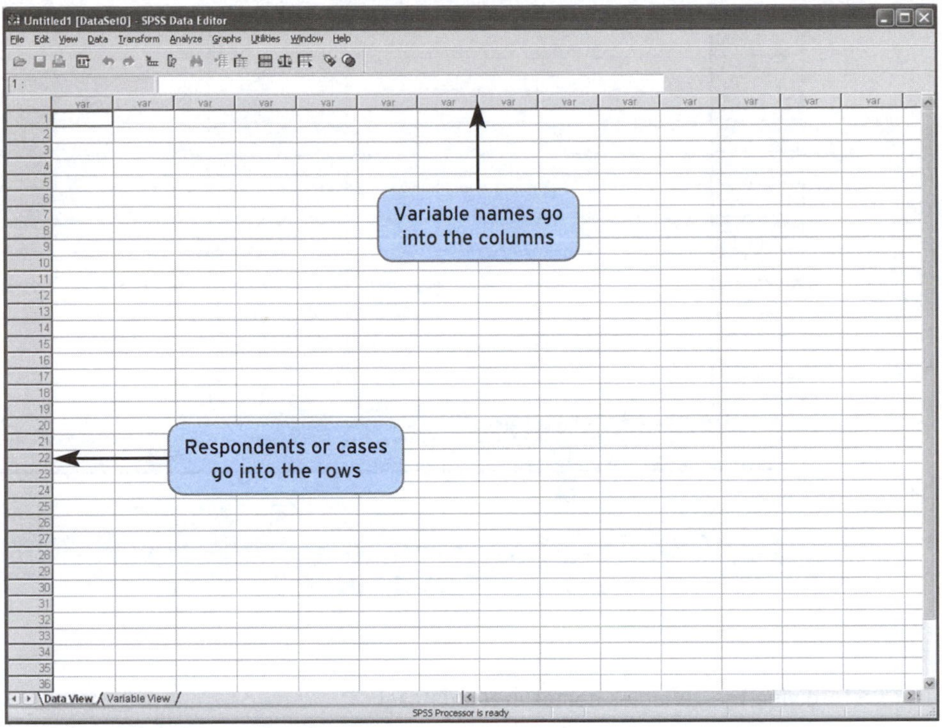

Figure 2.6 The SPSS data editor

PATIENT ANXIETY QUESTIONNAIRE

Please answer these questions by circling the appropriate response or filling in the gap.

Question 1. Sex: Male   Female

Question 2. What age are you?_____

Question 3. How anxious would you describe yourself in hospital situations?

[1] Not at all   [2] A little   [3] Not certain   [4] Quite a lot   [5] A lot

Figure 2.7 The patient anxiety questionnaire

Respondent 1	Respondent 2	Respondent 3	Respondent 4	Respondent 5
Q1. Male	Q1. Female	Q1. Female	Q1. Male	Q1. Male
Q2. 25	Q2. 27	Q2. 33	Q2. 29	Q2. 21
Q3. A little	Q3. Not at all	Q3. A lot	Q3. Not certain	Q3. A lot

Figure 2.8 Breakdown of responses to the patient anxiety questionnaire

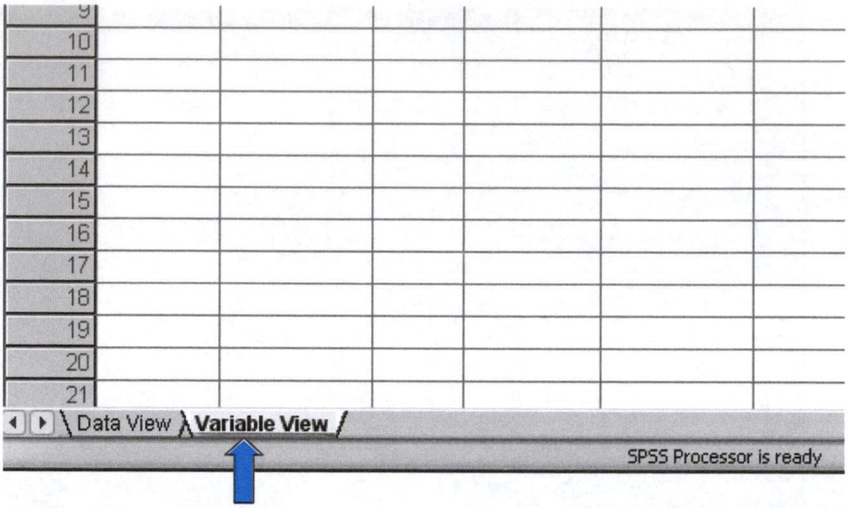

Figure 2.9 *The Variable View tab*

1 giving the variables names in the dataset;

2 giving the variables labels;

3 if appropriate, identifying what the level means for each variable;

4 identifying missing values.

Open SPSS. On the front datasheet, click on the **Variable View** tab in the bottom left-hand corner (Figure 2.9).

You are now in the sheet that allows you to enter information about each of your variables. It is slightly different on this sheet because the variables are now represented in the rows, rather than the columns in the Data View sheet. The columns now represent information about each of the variables.

Although there are many columns here we are interested only in using four of these columns: (1) **Name**, (2) **Label**, (3) **Values** and (4) **Missing**. We have indicated on Figure 2.10 how each column corresponds to each of the four stages mentioned above.

Variable names (column 1 of Figure 2.10)

Within SPSS for Windows we can name each variable. The variable name by convention is short (up to eight characters) and is used to remind you which variable each column represents. However, in later versions of SPSS for Windows, and unless you're using an older version of SPSS for Windows, variable names can be as a long as they need to be;

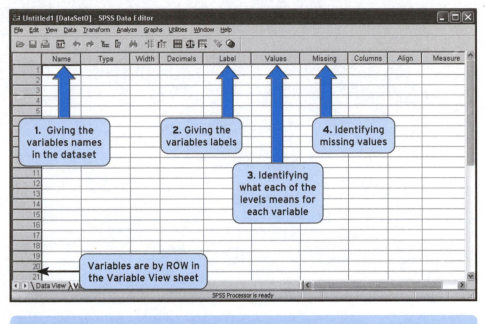

Figure 2.10 *The Variable View data grid*

they are just not allowed to contain any spaces (for example, use **variablename** rather than **variable name**).

Giving variable names to our variables above is fairly straightforward for the first two variables, sex and age of respondents. However, the name of our third variable, the level of patient anxiety of respondents, is longer than eight letters and so we need to abbreviate it. On this occasion it is fairly simple. We could just call the variable **anxiety**. For the future, it is useful to know that, in addition to not allowing spaces between words when creating a variable name, SPSS will not allow certain characters, such as @ and #, either.

To type in our variable names, all you do is type the variable names in the **Name** column, with each row representing a different variable (Figure 2.11). Here, type **sex**, **age** and **anxiety** into the first three rows of the first column. After you have typed in each word, press the arrow keys to move into the next box. Here, it will be the down-arrow key each time (alternatively you can position the cursor using the mouse).

Labelling each variable (column 2 of Figure 2.10)

Variable names are sometime confusing and you can forget what the shorter variable names mean. You can expand the detail of what the variable refers to in the **Label** column. All you can do in here is type in a fuller description. For example in Figure 2.12 we

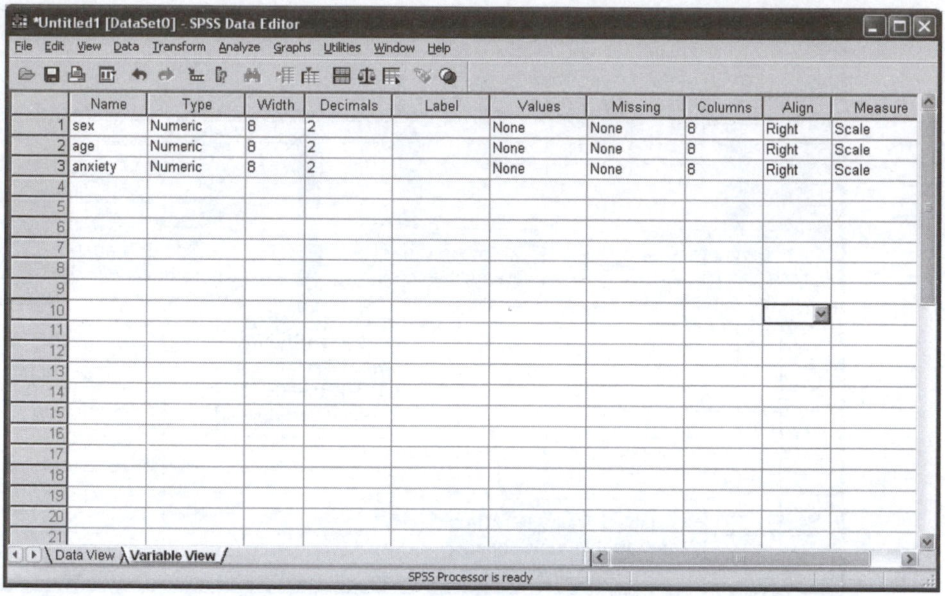

Figure 2.11 *Variable View window: entering variable names*

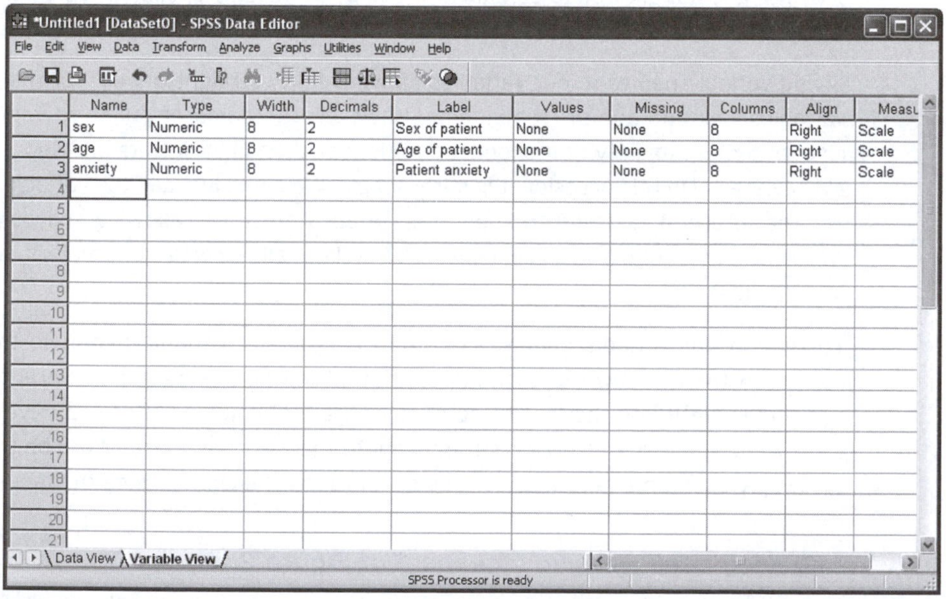

Figure 2.12 *Variable View window: labelling variables*

have simply typed in a fuller description for the sex (Sex of patient), age (Age of patient) and anxiety (Patient anxiety).

There is no need for you to do this, but it is considered good practice. This is because you may be working with a large dataset over a number of weeks and forget what all these shortened names mean. Or it may be that someone else wants to use your dataset, and rather than explain the names to them, all the information is there for them.

Therefore why don't you now just type these decriptions into the **Label** column for each variable.

Values for each level of the variables (column 3 of Figure 2.10)

For each variable, numerical values are assigned to each level. For some of your data you don't need to be reminded what each level means. For example, for age you will be able to remember that each number represents years. However, for other variables where you have assigned numbers (for example, where we have done it for sex of a respondent: 1 = Male, 2 = Female) it is useful to record these on the datasheet. To do this in SPSS for Windows, click on the box under **Values** that corresponds to the variable you wish to label, and then click on the grey section that appears (Figure 2.13).

You should now have a box that looks like that in Figure 2.14.

Here, for variable **sex**:

● Type **1** into the **Value:** box (for the first level).
● Type **Male** into the **Value Label:** box.

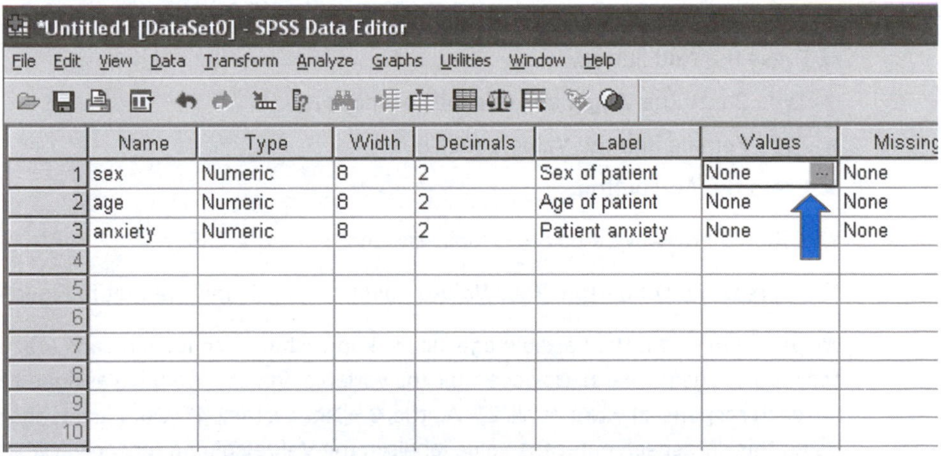

Figure 2.13 Close-up of the variables entered into the Variable View window

(a)

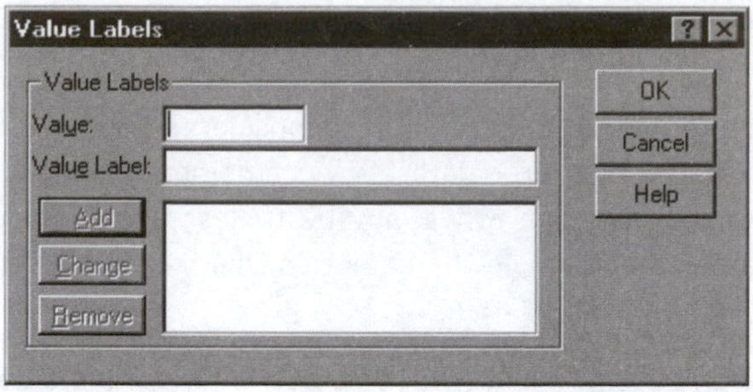

(b)

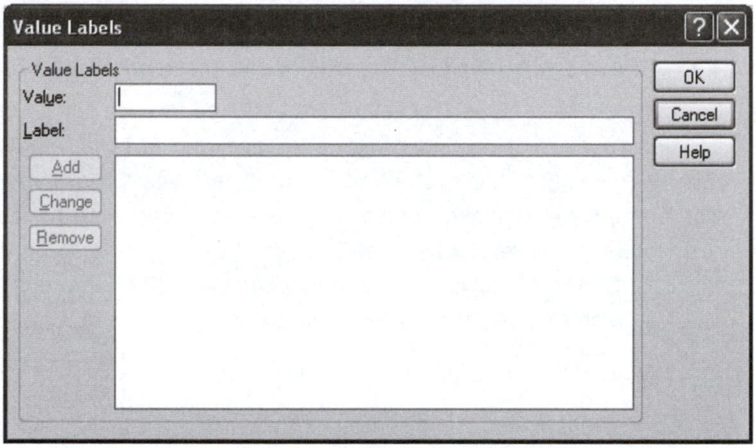

Figure 2.14 *Value Labels window. (a) Layout in older versions of SPSS for Windows. (b) Layout in newer versions of SPSS for Windows*

- Press the **Add** button.
- Type **2** into the **Value:** box (for the second level).
- Type **Female** into the **Value Label:** box.
- Press the **Add** button.

You should now have a box that looks like that in Figure 2.15.

Then press the **OK** button. Your **Values** column should look like that in Figure 2.16.

We would miss out the variable **age**, as we know what each level means (each number represents age in years). However, for the variable **anxiety**, we have assigned a number for each response: 1 = Not at all, 2 = A little, 3 = Not certain, 4 = Quite a lot, and 5 = A lot. Using this datasheet, enter the value labels in the **Value** column for the variable **anxiety**.

If you want to check whether you have entered this correctly, go to the book's website at **www.pearsoned.co.uk/maltby** where a correct version is presented.

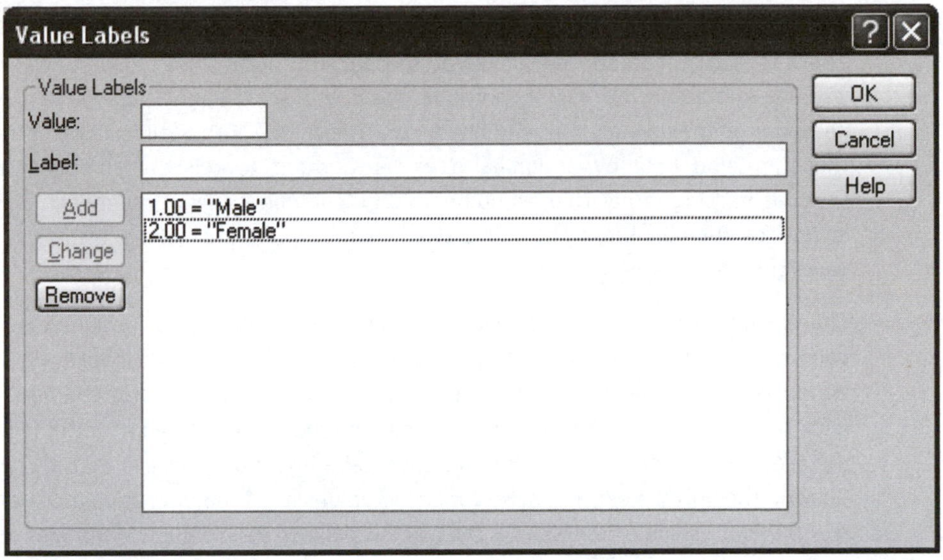

Figure 2.15 *Value Labels window with our Value Labels input*

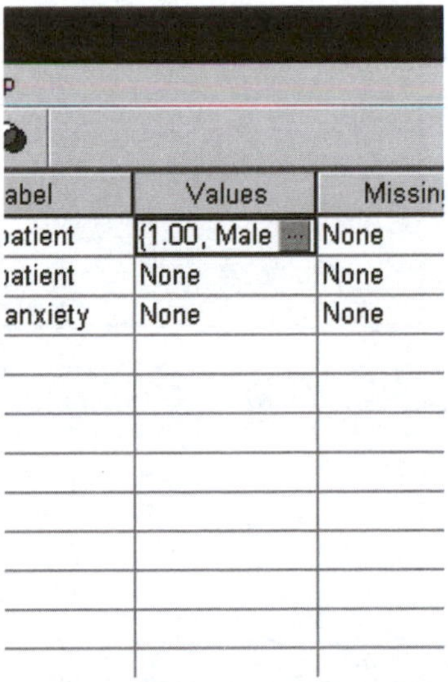

Figure 2.16 *A completed* **Values** *box*

Missing values (column 4 of Figure 2.10)

There is also a procedure to allow you to deal with data when people have not given you the required information, perhaps because they thought the question was too personal or they simply missed it by error. Either way, SPSS allows you to deal with these missing data by assigning a value to them to tell the computer to treat them as missing rather than as numbers. You can choose what number you assign to it, but traditionally the number 9 is used with single-figure values, or, if 9 is already used, then 99 or 999.

There is no need to enter these data with the current data because we have no missing values. However, if you want to practise, this is fairly straightforward. In SPSS for Windows, it is similar to labelling. Let us assign a missing value for the variable **sex**. Click on the box under **Missing** that corresponds to the variable **sex** and then click on the grey section that appears. You will then get a box that looks like that in Figure 2.17. Click on the button next to <u>D</u>iscrete missing values and type in your values. Here we've put in 9, but as you can see, SPSS for Windows allows you to put in a number of values, or in the row below a range of values (these options can be used for advanced options). You then press **OK**. You should now see a 9 under the missing column in the sex variable row. Now, when you have to allocate a value to a missing response to the sex item, you just type in 9 and the computer will ignore it.

Missing Values

- ○ <u>N</u>o missing values
- ◉ <u>D</u>iscrete missing values

  9

- ○ <u>R</u>ange plus one optional discrete missing value

  Low: High:

  Discrete value:

OK

Cancel

Help

Figure 2.17 *Missing Values window*

Exercise

1   Repeat this procedure for the variable **anxiety**.

2   Imagine some respondents did not want to reveal their age to you. What number would you assign as a missing value?

Putting your data into SPSS for Windows

Now we are going to put in the data. To move from the Variable View data window to the Data View window, press the **Data View** button in the bottom left-hand corner. Notice how the first three columns all have variable names. Now you can start putting in your data. Remember the patient anxiety questionnaire (Figure 2.18) and responses (Figure 2.19).

PATIENT ANXIETY QUESTIONNAIRE

Please answer these questions by circling the appropriate response or filling in the gap.

Question 1. Sex: Male   Female

Question 2. What age are you?_____

Question 3. How anxious would you describe yourself in hospital situations?

        [1] Not at all   [2] A little   [3] Not certain   [4] Quite a lot   [5] A lot

---

Figure 2.18 *The patient anxiety questionnaire*

Respondent 1	Respondent 2	Respondent 3	Respondent 4	Respondent 5
Q1. Male	Q1. Female	Q1. Female	Q1. Male	Q1. Male
Q2. 25	Q2. 27	Q2. 33	Q2. 29	Q2. 21
Q3. A little	Q3. Not at all	Q3. A lot	Q3. Not certain	Q3. A lot

---

Figure 2.19 *Breakdown of responses to the patient anxiety questionnaire*

Remember how you presented the data in the paper example. It is exactly the same as that. For the first row (respondent 1) you would put in **1** in the first column, **25** in the second column and **2** (A little) in the third column (Figure 2.20).

Exercise: Entering data in SPSS for Windows

Now continue entering data for each respondent. The completed dataset is on the website at **www.pearsoned.co.uk/maltby,** so you can check your results after you have had a go.

Finally, when you have finished inputting your data you will want to save the data. Box 2.7 tells you how to do this in SPSS.

Box 2.7 Task
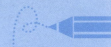

Saving data in SPSS for Windows

When you have finished inputting your data into SPSS, you will want to save the data. Whether you save the data on to your hard drive, floppy disk, your drive space at university or USB pen drive will depend on whether you are at home or at college. However, it is the same as saving a Word file (or anything else on the computer). Bring down the **File** menu and select the **Save As** option. A window entitled Newdata: Save Data As (see below) will open up. Choose where you want to save the data, be it on a floppy disk, hard drive, network space or USB pen drive, by exploring the **Save in:** box.

Save Data As window

When you have determined where you would like to save the file, type the file name (here, anxiety) in the **File name** box and then hit the **Save** button. Ensure that as you work and change a file, you keep saving it. As you know, computers can crash and if you are putting in a lot of data, nothing is more disheartening than to lose your work. So, as with all computer work, constantly save your file. And, if necessary, make a back-up.

Introduction to the book's datasets

Now you have learnt how to enter data into SPSS, we will be working with datasets that have been created for you. You will be able to conduct a variety of statistical tests

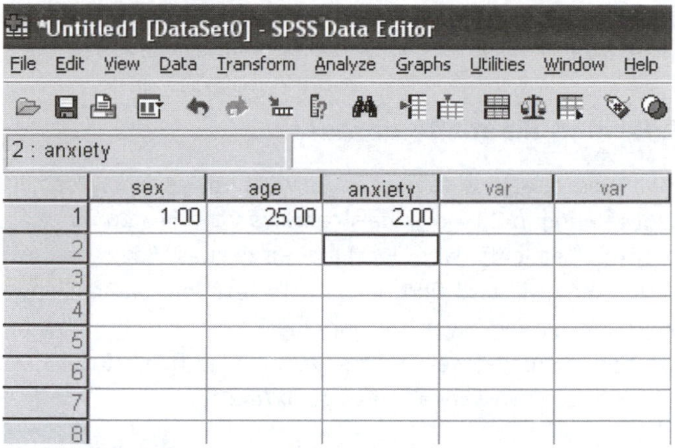

Figure 2.20 *Data that have been input from the patient anxiety questionnaire*

by using some of the lessons outlined in the following chapters in this book. There are five datasets that you can access. They are available on the accompanying website at **www.pearsoned.co.uk/maltby**.

Each of the datasets deals with subject matter relevant to nursing, and four of them in particular deal with the four major nursing branches, namely adult, mental health, child and learning disability nursing. Although these are hypothetical datasets, they are dealing with areas of primary interest to nurses.

● Adult branch dataset

The adult branch dataset is concerned with issues in adult branch nursing. In these data there are variables relating to 74 adults aged between 62 and 90 years. Variables in this dataset relate to prevention and management of falls among older people, issues of mobility and dementia, decision making and well-being. A full description of the dataset and the variables in the dataset itself are provided on the book's website at **www.pearsoned.co.uk/maltby**.

● Mental health dataset

The mental health dataset might be best used by mental health branch nurses. In this dataset you have been given details about a group of patients who have been diagnosed with schizophrenia. The dataset includes data on the use of atypical antipsychotic medication to prevent psychotic symptoms among these patients, data on treatment sessions and recovery and other aspects of provision carried out by the mental health nursing team. A full description of the dataset and the variables in the dataset itself are provided on the website at **www.pearsoned.co.uk/maltby**.

● Learning disability dataset

The learning disability dataset is relevant to learning disability branch nurses. This dataset relating to 24 individuals contains variables on the types of health and ability checks that patients with learning disabilities have had within general practice surgeries. You will also find out how to test for relationships between the patients' severity of learning disability and the health checks they have undergone. A full description of the dataset and the variables in the dataset itself are provided on the book's website at **www.pearsoned.co.uk/maltby**.

● Child branch dataset

The child branch dataset is useful for child branch nurses. It describes data collected in a survey of 40 mothers which looked at a number of factors around their giving birth in the previous year. In this dataset you can look at questions concerning: (1) parents' attitudes about the MMR vaccine and any intention to have their children vaccinated with the MMR jab; (2) their child's health; and (3) symptoms of post-natal depression. A full description of the dataset and the variables in the dataset itself are provided on the book's website at **www.pearsoned.co.uk/maltby**.

● MRSA dataset

The MRSA dataset regards data you will use in Chapter 6. It contains data regarding a number of hospitals' efforts to combat the MRSA hospital superbug via information packs on infection control and prevention given to staff, and leaflets and posters aimed at raising patients' and visitors' awareness of the problem. You will be introduced to this dataset in Chapter 6, but full details are available on the book's website at **www.pearsoned.co.uk/maltby**.

✚ Summary

In this chapter we have emphasised the central role of variables. Therefore, you should now be able to:

✔ **outline what variables are and how they are evident in many aspects of investigation;**

✔ **describe how variables are viewed by researchers;**

✔ **demonstrate the form variables take in SPSS for Windows by way of creating a datafile;**

✔ **use SPSS for Windows to create and save a datafile of variables.**

In the next chapter we are going to look at some of the ways that you can you use SPSS for Windows to describe variables.

Self-assessment exercise

In this exercise, we are going to give you just a light task. The exercise is designed to get you familiar with at least one of the aforementioned datasets. Go online to www.pearsoned.co.uk/maltby and download the datasets on to your hard drive or on to a disk so you have them readily available for when you are reading the subsequent chapters. We also suggest that you pick a couple of datasets, load them up on SPSS and look at some of the variables.

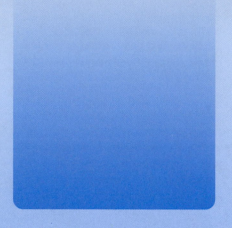

Chapter 3

Descriptive statistics: the Florence Nightingale way

Key themes

✔ Descriptive statistics

✔ Averages: mean, mode and median

✔ Variability, range, semi-interquartile range and standard deviation

✔ Recoding and computing variables

Learning outcomes

By the end of this chapter you will be able to:

✔ Demonstrate knowledge of frequency counts, averages, a measure of dispersion, bar charts and histograms, and how to perform these statistics on SPSS for Windows

✔ Perform in SPSS for Windows techniques in statistics that allow you to alter the structure of your data: the Recode and Compute commands

Introduction

Imagine . . . That you are an occupational health nurse working for a hospital employing over 400 nurses. Over the past few weeks, you have had several nurses who have been referred to your department with chronic back pain. This is a problem as it is unlikely that some of these nurses will be able to return to work and there are the human costs to these nurses' well-being and their worries about ever being able to work as a nurse again. You wonder whether there are system-related issues about how nurses are moving and handling patients in the wards. Are some nurses failing to use slides or hoists when moving patients? Are some nurses susceptible to taking short-cuts when moving and handling? You want to see how common these practices could be within the hospital and so you and your colleagues have decided to survey a sample of nurses to find out their attitudes towards adopting short-cuts to moving and handling and whether some nurses admit to doing so. You want to see whether there are any patterns among the nursing staff that are cause for concern: is it one in five nurses who take short-cuts when moving and handling or is it as many as one in three? Have more than half of the nurses surveyed said that they experience moderate to severe back pain when moving and handling patients? All of these figures are what is known as descriptive statistics and can help guide your decisions in your clinical practice.

One well-known nurse who used descriptive statistics to a positive end was Florence Nightingale. Although she is most renowned for being a pioneer of nursing and a reformer of hospital sanitation methods, her use of descriptive statistics played a part in such reforms. **Descriptive statistics** are techniques to collect, organise, interpret and make graphical displays of information. It was techniques such as this that allowed Florence Nightingale to outline the incidence of preventable deaths through unsanitary conditions in the army during the Crimean War and helped her to lead the way to sanitation reform.

In this chapter we introduce you to descriptive statistics, and, more specifically, frequency counts, averages, a measure of dispersion, bar charts and histograms. We also introduce you to a couple of techniques in statistics that allow you to alter the structure of your data, the 'recode' and 'compute' statements.

Energiser

Before you start, we are going to get your brain warmed up mathematically, and get you to carry out some simple calculations. These calculations are related to some of the concepts you will come across in the chapter.

1 For each set of numbers, add together the numbers.

   (a) 4, 3, 2, 1, 5

   (b) 3, 2, 1, 2, 5

2 For each set of numbers, rank the numbers in ascending (lowest to highest) order.

   (a) 7, 5, 2, 4, 3, 9, 17

   (b) 2, 7, 62, 53, 1, 2

3 For each set of numbers, rank the numbers in descending (highest to lowest) order.

   (a) 15, 5, 12, 4, 31, 9, 17

   (b) 23, 7, 2, 53, 11, 2

4 For each set of numbers, rank the numbers in ascending order. What is the middle number?

   (a) 1, 9, 5, 4, 3, 2, 8

   (b) 19, 13, 17, 18, 12, 21, 23

5 For each set of numbers, which is the most frequent number?

   (a) 2, 56, 3, 3, 2, 2, 13, 23

   (b) 117, 112, 113, 117, 119

6 For each set of numbers, (i) add together the numbers in each set, and (ii) count how many numbers are in each set. Then divide your answer for (i) by your answer for (ii).

   (a) 1, 7, 6, 3, 3, 4

   (b) 23, 27, 18, 12, 20

The above calculations actually refer to some of the statistics you are going to read about in this chapter.

Descriptive statistics: describing variables

In nursing we are surrounded by statistics. For example, the BBC News health website (www.bbc.co.uk/health) and the *Nursing Times* website (www.nursingtimes.net/) list the following facts:

- Smoking is the single largest cause of preventable cancer deaths in the UK. On average, each year it causes 32,000 deaths from lung cancer and 11,000 deaths from other cancers.

- On average, nearly one in four British women dies as a result of heart disease. Women who have a heart attack are less likely than men to survive the initial event.

- Around 40 to 50 per cent of women diagnosed with ovarian cancer will still be alive five years later. When the disease is caught early, however, survival rates are much higher, although the particular type and severity of the cancer are also important factors.

- The Population Reference Bureau (2004) suggests that there will be a total of 10.5 million older people in the UK (16 per cent of the population) by 2050.

- It is estimated that there are about 338,000 new cases of angina pectoris (a common, disabling, chronic cardiac condition) per year in the UK (British Heart Foundation, 2004).

As we mentioned at the beginning of the book, we constantly use statistics, particularly the statistics addressed in this chapter of the book. We know how much of our income we spend on different things, for example how much on rent/mortgage payments, how much on food, how much on clothes. You would also be able to estimate what percentage you spend on these things, and if not, you could say that you spent a greater percentage of your income per month on your rent/mortgage than on clothes. We know roughly, on average, how much a week we spend (or can afford). We know the average house prices on the street where we live. In your profession, you will be continually presented with statistical descriptive data: mortality rates, average life expectancy, percentage recovery rate, average remission time. Most of your job, treatment strategies, policies that surround your job, and all these facts described above are derived from the use of descriptive statistics.

All the statistics we mentioned above are ways of describing things: how much you work, how much your mortgage is, what mortality rates are, what effective treatment strategies are. Therefore, you wouldn't be surprised to find out that descriptive statistics are simply ways of describing data. There are many different types of descriptive statistics, but the aim of this book is to teach the most used and relevant statistics. Using these criteria, teaching descriptive statistics becomes fairly directed, and you will find, in most journal articles, that these are the main statistics that researchers use.

There are four main areas of descriptive statistics that we will cover. These are:

- frequencies
- averages
- charts
- variability.

Frequencies

The first aspect is frequencies of data. This information can be used to break down any variable and to tell the researcher how many respondents answered at each level of the variable. Consider an example where a hospital administrator is deciding whether to carry out an awareness scheme in his hospital of the causes of back pain in nurses while carrying out their daily duties (including heavy lifting, lifting patients correctly). He asked 100 nurses working in the hospital whether they had experienced any back

Table 3.1 Answers to the question 'Have you experienced back pain?'

Possible answer	Frequency of answer
Severe	7 respondents answered the question with this response
Minor	45 respondents answered the question with this response
None	48 respondents answered the question with this response

pain in the past six months. Respondents were given three choices of answer: 1 = Severe, 2 = Minor, and 3 = None. To examine the prevalence of back pain among nurses, the administrator adds up the number of responses to each of the possible answers, and presents them in a table in order to examine the frequency of answers to each possible response (see Table 3.1).

On this occasion seven respondents said they had experienced severe back pain, 45 respondents said they had experienced minor back pain and 48 respondents said they experienced no back pain. As we can see, almost half of the nurses had suffered some sort of back pain, and as the occupational health nurse with responsibilities for back care in the hospital you may be concerned about this finding.

This type of breakdown of answers is how frequencies of information are determined. Frequencies refer to the number of times something is found. In statistics, frequencies are most often presented in the form of a **frequency table**, similar to Table 3.1.

● Frequencies on SPSS for Windows

We are now going to show you how to obtain frequencies on SPSS for Windows. In the following examples we are going to use data from the learning disabilities dataset. In this dataset there are 20 questions relating to 24 people diagnosed as having learning difficulties. Questions included in this dataset refer to the sex of the person with the learning disability, their age, their type of learning disability, and the number of consultations the person has had with the learning disability nurse.

First, we are going to obtain the frequencies for one variable in the dataset: the type of learning disability (a categorical-type variable - remember, a categorical-type variable is one that is made up of different and separate categories). Load up the dataset. We are going to produce a frequency table for the variable **Diagnosi** / Diagnosis for Learning Disability (fifth variable down in the list), the type of learning disability the person has. Click on the **Analyze** pull-down menu. Click on **Descriptive Statistics** and pull the mouse over to **Frequencies** and click on this. You will get a screen that looks like Figure 3.1.

Move the variable **Diagnosi** from the left-hand box into the **Variable(s):** box by using the arrow button. Then hit **OK**. You should get a table like that in Figure 3.2 as a new screen

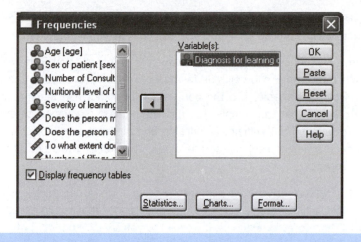

Figure 3.1 *SPSS screen for frequencies*

Diagnosis for learning disability

		Frequency	Percent	Valid Percent	Cumulative Percent
Valid	Arrested hydrocephaly	1	4.2	4.2	4.2
	Birth trauma	3	12.5	12.5	16.7
	Brain damage	2	8.3	8.3	25.0
	Brain damage RTA	1	4.2	4.2	29.2
	Cerebral palsy	1	4.2	4.2	33.3
	Chickenpox encephalitis	1	4.2	4.2	37.5
	Congenital abnormality	1	4.2	4.2	41.7
	Down's syndrome	6	25.0	25.0	66.7
	Dysgenic features	1	4.2	4.2	70.8
	Microcephaly	2	8.3	8.3	79.2
	Multiple handicap at birth	1	4.2	4.2	83.3
	Not recorded	1	4.2	4.2	87.5
	Williams' syndrome	3	12.5	12.5	100.0
	Total	24	100.0	100.0	

Figure 3.2 *Frequencies of diagnosis for learning disability*

appears. This is called the output window (this is where all your output from SPSS appears and you can save, edit and print this as you would a Word file).

In this frequency table we can get two sets of information from the first two columns (ignore the other two columns for now). We are interested in the frequency of each level of the variable, and the percentage breakdown of each level. In this example we can see that the sample that has the highest frequency is for Down's syndrome (six reports), then Williams' syndrome and birth trauma (both three), and then brain damage and microcephaly (both two), and then for all the other diagnoses there is only one report.

This table also gives you a percentage breakdown. A percentage is the proportion of a variable falling within a certain value or category that is expressed in terms of 'out of 100'. Therefore, for example, if we said to you that 80 per cent of patients were happy with the care they received in hospital, you would know that the majority of patients were happy about their standard of care. If we said to you 80 patients were happy with the care they received in hospital, your first question would be 'How many people did you ask?' (If we had asked 80, then great; but if we had asked 80,000, then perhaps not so great.) Therefore, percentages are a descriptive statistic that allow us to quickly summarise and put some meaning behind our findings. In percentage terms, 25 per cent of our sample has been diagnosed with Down's syndrome.

Averages

Consider the following findings from published articles, noting when the term *average* is used.

Article 1

A study carried out by McEwen *et al.* (2005) to investigate the self-reported duties performed by sisters and charge nurses working on the wards reported the following findings:

- Sisters/charge nurses reported directly assessing on *average* 75 per cent of patients on their ward during a typical shift.
- Sisters/charge nurses were allocated patients for whom they had not planned to take primary responsibility in addition to being in charge of the ward a mean average of 2.5 shifts per week.
- On *average* they reported spending almost six hours a week outside of their contracted hours on ward business.

Article 2

Marshall *et al.* (2005) reported on a study which sought to reduce waiting times for a rapid-access chest pain clinic (RACPC). Between March and October 2003, patients referred to the RACPC waited an *average* of 34 days for an appointment. There was a high proportion of inappropriate referrals to the clinic. As part of a review of strategy, Marshall and her colleagues oversaw a service redesign, and a process-mapping session was conducted in which key players in the patient's journey informed each other of how their work was interrelated. As a result of the above changes, the team achieved, and sustained, a 14-day waiting target for the clinic, with the current *average* wait down to 8 days.

You have probably heard or read the phrase 'on average' a lot throughout your life, and probably many times during your time in nursing. Averages are ways in which researchers can summarise frequency data and find out what are the most common responses. Both the above articles use averages to describe a situation or event. Article 1 uses averages to indicate the amount of time spent by sisters and charge nurses on their duties. Article 2 uses averages to show falls in waiting times for a rapid-access chest pain clinic.

There are three types of average, known as the mean, the mode and the median.

- **Mean.** This is calculated by adding together all the values from each response to the variable, and dividing by the number of respondents.
- **Median.** This is calculated by putting all the values from responses to the variable in order, from the smallest value to the largest value, and selecting the value that appears in the middle.
- **Mode.** This is the value that occurs most often in the set of data.

Consider this example. A doctor wants to assess quickly how long patients wait in the hospital's emergency ward before they are seen. The researcher collates the information into frequencies, and displays the data in the form of a table (Table 3.2).

The researcher wishes to work out the mean, median and mode.

For the *mean* the researcher adds all the responses, 10 + 10 + 10 + 20 + 60 (three patients had to wait 10 minutes, one patient had to wait 20 minutes, and one patient had to wait 60 minutes) and divides the total 110 (10 + 10 + 10 + 20 + 60 = 110) by the number of respondents asked. Here, five patients took part in the research, so 110 is divided by 5. Therefore, the mean equals 110 divided by 5, which is 22. Therefore, there is a mean of 22 minutes before people are seen.

Table 3.2 Answers to the question 'How long did you have to wait before being seen?'

Possible answer	Frequency of answer
10 minutes	3 patients
20 minutes	1 patient
30 minutes	
40 minutes	
50 minutes	
60 minutes	1 patient
...	

For the *median*, you choose the middle number from all the numbers presented in numerical order. So, rank the numbers from the smallest to the highest, 10, 10, 10, 20, 60, and then select the middle number, which is 10. Therefore, there is a median of 10 minutes' waiting time. This is fairly straightforward when the researcher has an odd number of cases. When there is an even number, you select the middle two numbers and divide their sum by 2. So in the case of having four waiting times, say 10, 10, 20 and 60, you would add together 10 and 20 and divide by 2, giving 30 divided by 2 which equals 15. The median waiting time is 15 minutes.

For the *mode*, the most common number is selected. In the example, 10, 10, 10, 20, 60, the most common number is 10, so 10 is the mode. Therefore, there is a mode of 10 minutes' waiting time in the hospital.

Therefore, the researcher will report that among his sample the mean average waiting time for the five patients is 22 minutes, the median waiting time is 10 minutes and the mode waiting time is 10 minutes.

However, it is not common practice to report all three measures of average. Rather, the mean is the most commonly used, and as a rule the median and the mode tend to be used only when researchers suspect that reporting the mean may not represent a fair summary of the data. For example, in the case above, perhaps reporting a mean waiting time of 22 minutes would be unfair to the staff working in the ward. A much fairer assessment would be to use the median and mode because they seem to reflect more accurately the average of 10 minutes, particularly as all but one patient is seen in under 22 minutes.

In terms of statistics, it is sometimes best to use the mean and sometimes best to use the median. Throughout the rest of this book we will point out when (and why) it is best to use the mean and when (and why) it is best to use the median.

● Obtaining averages on SPSS for Windows

We are now going to show you how to obtain averages on SPSS for Windows. In the following examples we are going, again, to use data from the learning disabilities dataset.

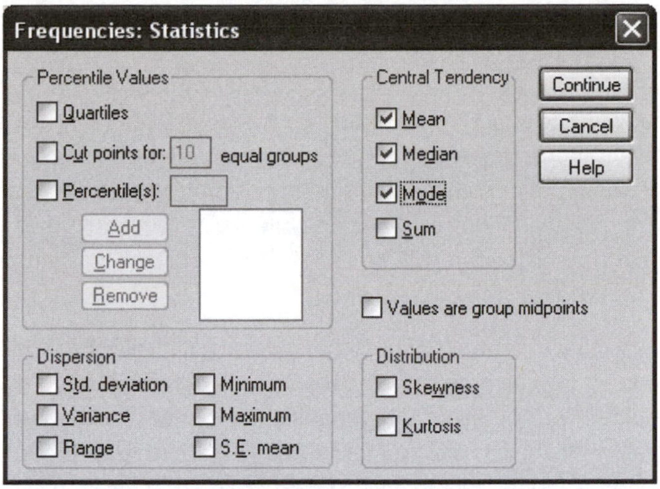

Figure 3.3 *Frequencies: Statistics window*

In this dataset there are a number of questions relating to 24 people diagnosed as having learning difficulties, including regarding their sex, age and the type of learning difficulty.

We are going to obtain the averages for one variable in the dataset: the number of consultations the individual has had with the learning disability nurse, [**consulta**] (this is a continuous-type variable).

To get the average statistics for this variable, pull down the **Analyze** menu, click on **Descriptive Statistics**, then pull the mouse over to **Frequencies**, and click on this. The screen will look similar to the previous one for frequencies. Transfer the variable [**consulta**] / Number of Consultations (third variable down) into the **Variable(s):** box using the arrow button. However, before pressing **OK**, click on the **Statistics...** box at the bottom of the window. The screen will look like that in Figure 3.3. Click in the boxes next to **Mean**, **Median** and **Mode** under **Central Tendency**.

Now click on **Continue** and then **OK**. You will get a figure that looks like Figure 3.4.

As you can see, the mean is 9.83, the median is 8 and the mode is 8.

N	Valid	24
	Missing	0
Mean		9.83
Median		8.00
Mode		8(a)

Figure 3.4 *Mean, median and mode of number of consultations with learning disability nurse*

Charts: visual presentation of your data

On SPSS for Windows you can also provide graphical representations of variables. One advantage of descriptive statistics is that you can carry out a number of graphical representations. However, it is often a temptation to become overinvolved with graphs. We are going to concentrate on the three simple graphs (the bar chart, the histogram and the pie chart), not only because they are frequently used but also because one of them (the histogram) will be used as an important building block in understanding further statistics in the next chapter.

All these charts are ways of presenting data graphically. Bar charts and pie charts tend to be used for categorical-type data, and histograms tend to be used for continuous-type data. We will, using the variables mentioned above (Type of Learning Disability [categorical-type] and Number of Consultations with the learning disability nurse [continuous-type]), show you how to obtain bar charts, pie charts and histograms on SPSS.

● Obtaining a bar chart on SPSS for Windows

A **bar chart** is a chart with rectangular bars of lengths that represent the frequencies of each aspect and is mainly used for categorical-type data (data which is made up of different categories). We can show this for the type of learning disability variable in the learning disability dataset. Pull down the **G**raphs menu, and click on **Bar..** and a new screen will appear. Click on **Simple**, and then **Define**. Move the variable **Diagnosi /** Diagnosis for Learning Disability into the **Category Ax̲is** and press **OK**. You will now see a chart like that in Figure 3.5.

The variable levels (type of learning disability) are plotted along the bottom (this is called the *x*-axis) and the frequency of each level is plotted up the side (this is called the *y*-axis). Notice how the bars are separate; this indicates that the variable is categorical-type.

● Obtaining a pie chart on SPSS for Windows

A **pie chart** is a circular chart divided into segments, illustrating the different frequencies, proportional to the size of the frequency to all the other frequencies (much in the same way as a percentage works). Florence Nightingale is credited with developing an early form of the pie chart and much of her work is credited to the fact that she was able to present her data in this way.

Let's get a pie chart for our type of learning disability variable. Pull down the **G**raphs menu and click on **Pie..** . A new screen will appear. Make sure the **Summaries for Groups of Cases** is selected (which it should be) and then click on **Define**. Move the variable

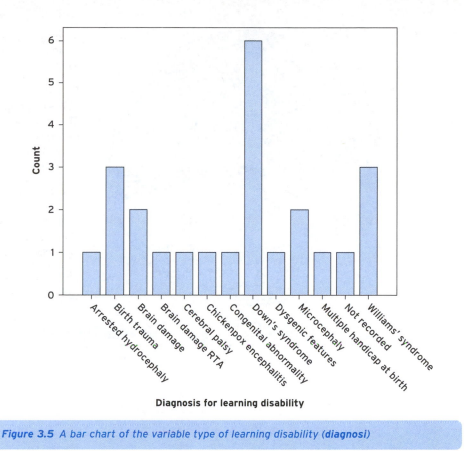

Figure 3.5 *A bar chart of the variable type of learning disability (**diagnosi**)*

Diagnosi / Diagnosis for Learning Disability into the **Define Slices By**, and press **OK**. You will now get a chart like that in Figure 3.6.

● Obtaining a histogram on SPSS for Windows

A **histogram** is a graphical display of the frequencies of a variable and is mainly used with continuous-type data (data comprising numbers in some numerical order). For this graph we are going to use the number of consultations the individual has had with the learning disability nurse.

Pull down the **Graphs** menu and click on **Histogram...**. A new screen will appear. Transfer the [**consulta**] / Number of Consultations variable into the **Variable(s):** box and hit **OK**. You will then get the output shown in Figure 3.7.

The variable levels (possible scores) are plotted along the *x*-axis and the frequency of each level is plotted along the *y*-axis). Notice how the bars are together, indicating that the variable is continuous-type.

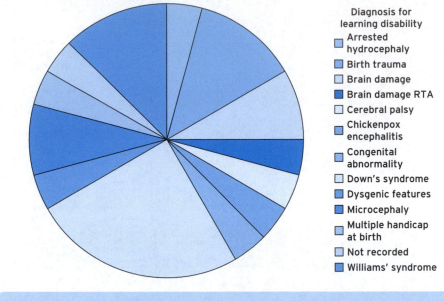

Figure 3.6 *A pie chart of the variable type of learning disability (**diagnosi**)*

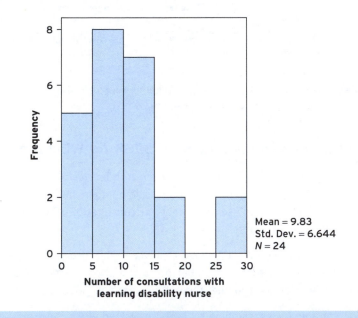

Mean = 9.83
Std. Dev. = 6.644
N = 24

Figure 3.7 *A histogram of the variable **number of consultations with learning disability nurse***

![brain icon] **Exercise: means and graphical representations in SPSS for Windows**

One of the variables in this dataset refers to the assessed severity of the learning disability (**severity**). 0 was not severe at all, whereas 100 was considered a profound severity. A midpoint of 50 was indicated to represent mild severity of learning disability. Work out the mean, median and mode of the variable Severity of learning disability (**severity**). Also choose which graphical representation you would use to display these data.

Variability

So far we have looked at averages (mean, median and mode) and charts (bar charts, pie charts and histograms). However, let us put the following to you. In Table 3.3 we present you with the average statistics of the average age of two sets of patients assigned to two charge nurses in a hospital: Charge Nurse Williams has 56 patients, and Charge Nurse Maltby also has 56 patients.

As you can see, the profile of the average statistics for the age of each set of patients (mean = 40, median = 40, mode = 40) suggests the two charge nurses are dealing with an identical set of patients (in terms of their age). Everything seems equitable.

However, let us look at these statistics again. Figure 3.8 shows a frequency table and histogram of the age of patients seen by Charge Nurse Williams. Figure 3.9 shows a frequency table and histogram of the age of patients seen by Charge Nurse Maltby. As you can see, the actual ages of each set of patients *vary* for each charge nurse. Charge Nurse Williams sees patients ranging from newborn babies to those aged 80 years, whereas Charge Nurse Maltby sees patients ranging in age from 30 years to 50 years. Therefore, their workload regarding the age range of the patients varies greatly.

This is an example of **variability**, that is, the extent to which scores within a particular sample vary. What we will show you now is the three ways that statisticians usually

Table 3.3 Mean age of patients by charge nurse

	Charge Nurse Williams	Charge Nurse Maltby
N Valid	56	56
Missing	0	0
Mean	40.0000	40.0000
Median	40.0000	40.0000
Mode	40.00	40.00

		Frequency	Percentage	Valid percentage	Cumulative percentage
Valid	0.00	2	3.6	3.6	3.6
	10.00	4	7.1	7.1	10.7
	20.00	5	8.9	8.9	19.6
	30.00	10	17.9	17.9	37.5
	40.00	14	25.0	25.0	62.5
	50.00	10	17.9	17.9	80.4
	60.00	5	8.9	8.9	89.3
	70.00	4	7.1	7.1	96.4
	80.00	2	3.6	3.6	100.0
	Total	56	100.0	100.0	

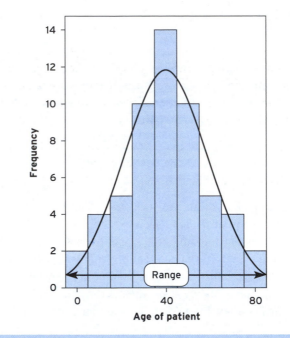

Figure 3.8 *Frequency table and histogram of the ages of patients seen by Charge Nurse Williams*

describe variability: through the use of (1) the range, (2) the semi-interquartile range and (3) the standard deviation.

Range

The first way that we show variability is by reporting the range of scores. So, for Charge Nurse Williams, his/her patients' ages range from 0 to 80, and therefore the **range** of scores is 80 (worked out by subtracting the smaller number from the larger number). Therefore, the range of scores for Charge Nurse Maltby is 20 (= 50 – 30).

		Frequency	Percentage	Valid percentage	Cumulative percentage
Valid	30.00	5	8.9	8.9	8.9
	35.00	13	23.2	23.2	32.1
	40.00	20	35.7	35.7	67.9
	45.00	13	23.2	23.2	91.1
	50.00	5	8.9	8.9	100.0
	Total	56	100.0	100.0	

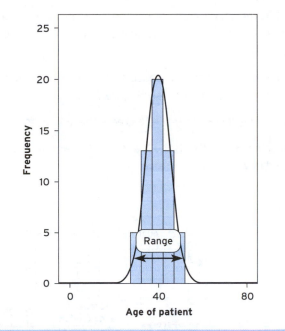

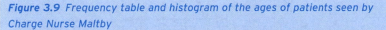

Figure 3.9 *Frequency table and histogram of the ages of patients seen by Charge Nurse Maltby*

We can now see that although the average age of all their patients is similar, the ages of Charge Nurse Williams' patients have a much greater range (range = 80) than Charge Nurse Maltby's (range = 20).

Therefore, you can see how the use of averages might also be presented with some indication of the variability of scores. You will see, in research studies that use average statistics, that some mention of the variability of scores is made.

However, the range is sometimes considered a rather oversimplified way of showing variability. This is because sometimes it may overemphasise extreme scores. Take, for example, another charge nurse, Charge Nurse Day, who has 100 patients; 99 of his/her patients are aged from 20 to 40 years, but there is one patient who is aged 80 years.

With that patient the age range is 60. Without this one patient aged 80, the age range is 20. Therefore, the presence of this one 80-year-old patient has distorted the range. Consequently, the range is sometimes considered an unreliable measure of variability, and you will see two other measures of variability more commonly used: the semi-interquartile range and the standard deviation.

● Semi-interquartile range (SIQR)

The **semi-interquartile range** is a descriptive statistic of variability that usually accompanies the use of the *median* average statistic (you see why when we describe the semi-interquartile range).

The semi-interquartile range is based on the idea that you can divide any distribution of scores into four equal parts (see Figure 3.10).

Three cuts – **quartiles** – are made to create these four equal parts. They are:

● *First quartile* – this cuts off the lowest 25 per cent of scores (at the 25th **percentile**). It is also known as the *lower quartile* or Q1.

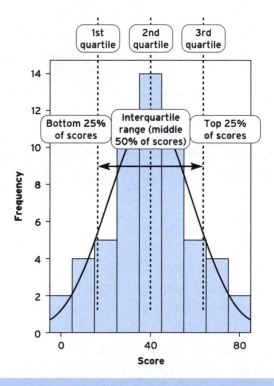

Figure 3.10 Quartile ranges of a set of scores

- *Second quartile* – this uses the median average (in other words, the 50th percentile score) to split the data in half. It is also known as Q2.
- *Third quartile* – this cuts off the highest 25 per cent of data, at the 75th percentile. It is also known as the *upper quartile* or Q3.

As you can see, we have four sections each representing 25 per cent of the scores (a quarter of the scores). You will have also seen that we have highlighted three sections, the bottom 25 per cent (those scores under the first quartile), the top 25 per cent (those scores over the third quartile) and the interquartile range, which are those scores between the first quartile (the bottom 25 per cent) and the third quartile (top 25 per cent). These are the basic ideas that underlie working out the semi-interquartile range.

To work out the semi-interquartile range, we first need to find out what the interquartile range is, and divide that into two (semi means half, as in semi-detached, semi-conscious).

This can be a little tricky to work out by hand so we are going to show you how to do it on SPSS first (Box 3.1 later in this chapter shows you how to work out a set of numbers by hand). Let us look at a variable in the learning disability dataset, Severity of Learning Disability (**severity**). Load up this dataset. In this dataset of 24 people with learning disabilities, each person has been rated on the severity of learning disability on a scale of 0 to 100, with higher scores indicating a greater degree of severity. To work out the semi-interquartile range, click on **Analyze**, then click on **Descriptive Statistics** and then **Frequencies**. You should then get a window that looks like that in Figure 3.11a. Then transfer **severity** into the **Variables(s):** box using the arrow button. Press the **Statistics** button and click the box next to **Quartiles** where it should now be ticked (see Figure 3.11b). Click on **Continue** and then **OK**. You should then get an output screen that looks like that in Figure 3.12.

In this figure you will recognise the frequency table (the second table), but it is the first table you are interested in. This table tells you the figure for the first quartile, the 25th percentile, which is equal to 25, and the third quartile, the 75th percentile, which is 80. Now, to work out the **interquartile range** (and similar to when working out the range), you subtract the lowest number (25) from the highest number (80), giving you 55. Therefore, your interquartile range is 55. And therefore, your semi-interquartile range is half of that, 55 divided by 2, which 27.5. So the semi-interquartile range is 27.5.

Therefore, the semi-interquartile range is another indicator of variability. As this indic-ator of variability relies on splitting the sample, in other words the second quartile division is based on a median split (i.e. the 50th percentile/halfway), you often find that when the median is used as an indicator of an average the semi-interquartile range is used as an indicator of variability.

(a)

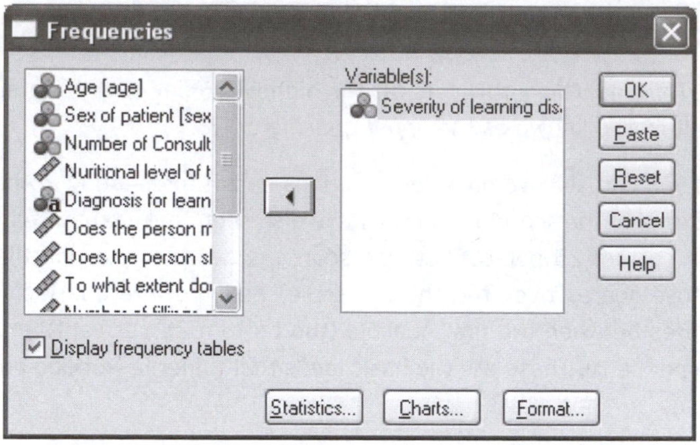

(b)

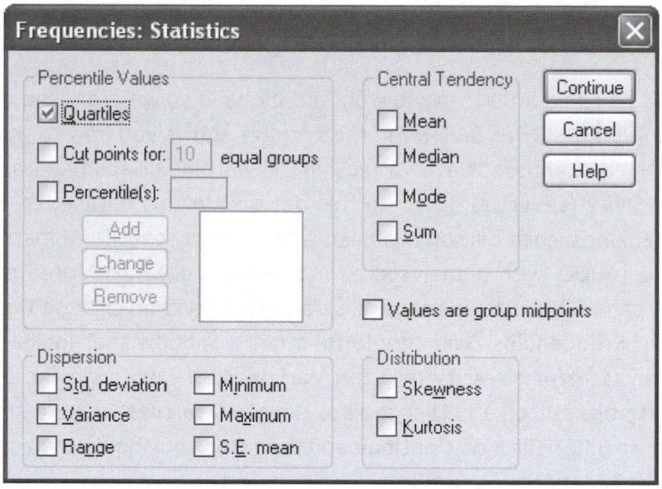

Figure 3.11 *Frequencies and Frequencies: Statistics windows*

● Standard deviation

Whereas the semi-interquartile range is a descriptive statistic of variability that accompanies the use of the median average statistic, the **standard deviation** is a descriptive statistic of variability that accompanies the use of the *mean* average statistic. Like the semi-interquartile range, the standard deviation provides the researcher with an indicator of how scores for variables are spread around the mean average (this is why it is sometimes referred to as a measure of dispersion).

Calculating the standard deviation is a little harder than calculating the semi-interquartile range so we are not going into detail; just remember that the standard

Statistics

Severity of learning disability

N	Valid	24
	Missing	0
Percentiles	25	25.00
	50	60.00
	75	80.00

Severity of learning disability

		Frequency	Percentage	Valid percentage	Cumulative percentage
Valid	20	6	25.0	25.0	25.0
	40	6	25.0	25.0	50.0
	80	11	45.8	45.8	95.8
	100	1	4.2	4.2	100.0
	Total	24	100.0	100.0	

Figure 3.12 SPSS output window (percentiles)

deviation provides the researcher with an indicator of how scores for variables are spread around the mean average (we have described how this can be done by hand in Box 3.1). However, we will now tell you how to get the standard deviation in SPSS for Windows.

Remember in the previous example where you clicked **Quartiles** under Learning Disability Severity. Well, you can get the standard deviation from the same Window. Return to the learning disability dataset and click on **Analyze**, then click on **Descriptive Statistics** and then **Frequencies**. **Severity** is already in the box (from last time); if not, transfer **severity** into the **Variables(s):** box using the arrow button. Now click on the **Statistics** button. Again, if you are continuing on from the previous section, **Quartiles** will still be ticked. If it is, click on the box next to it to remove the tick. To get the standard deviation for the severity of the learning disability, click the box next to **Std. deviation** under dispersion. Now click on **Continue** and then **OK**. You will then get an output like that in Figure 3.13. It is the first box we are interested in, and you will see that the standard deviation is 27.649.

But what does the number 27.649 mean? Sometimes it is hard to assess what all these measures of variability actually mean, but the higher the variability (that is, the higher the range, the semi-interquartile range or the standard deviation), the more that scores are spread out around the mean. Therefore, a higher variability would be found for a set of five scores comprising 0, 15, 55, 78, 100 (the standard deviation here is 41.93), than for a set comprising 1, 2, 2, 3, 4 (here the standard deviation is 1.13). Though on its own a variability can often seem redundant, it is useful when you are comparing two

Box 3.1 Point to consider

Working out the semi-interquartile range and standard deviation by hand

We are now going to develop your skills with using numbers by showing you how to work out the semi-interquartile range and the standard deviation by hand.

Calculating the semi-interquartile range by hand

If we wanted to find the semi-interquartile range for the following set of 11 numbers 1, 2, 5, 6, 7, 8, 11, 12, 18, 19, 31 (make sure your numbers are ordered from lowest to highest), we would do the following.

To work out the lower quartile, we would take the number of values (n, which stands for number of values in a sample), here 11, and add 1 (which is $n + 1$), which gives us 12.

Then, to work out the lower quartile we would divide ($n + 1$) by 4; so here it is 12 divided by 4, which is 3. Therefore we would take the third value, which in our case is 5. So the lower quartile is 5.

Then to work out the upper quartile we would multiply ($n + 1$) by 3 and then divide by 4. So this would be 12 multiplied by 3, and then divided by 4, which is 9. Therefore we would take the ninth value, which in our case is 18.

Then to work out the interquartile range we would take away 5 from 18, which is 13. To work out the semi-interquartile range we would then divide this result by 2, which is 13 divided by 2, which is 6.5. Therefore for the set of numbers above the **semi-interquartile range** = 6.5.

Note

As with the median, if you find when working out what number value you should pick, the calculation says you should take, say, the 3.5th value, select the two numbers that surround this number in your list and divide by 2. The resulting number will be your quartile. So if, for example, your calculation of the lower quartile was 3.5, suggesting you choose the 3.5th value in the following set of number 1, 3, 5, 6, 7, 8, 5, . . . , you should take 5 and 6 (the 3rd and 4th numbers) and divide by 2, which is 11 divided by 2, which is 5.5.

Calculating the standard deviation by hand

We are now going to develop your skills with statistics by showing you how to work out the standard deviation by hand. There are two formulae for working out the standard deviation. However, we are going to use the more common one. This is the standard deviation used with data from samples.

A researcher has decided to examine how much a sample of five people with learning disabilities vary in their visits to the learning disability nurse. He found out recently that in another ward the standard deviation of visits was 2.34. From the sample the researcher finds that the frequencies of visits of the five individuals over the past six months were 1, 3, 3, 4, 4. To work out the standard deviation the researcher would need to do the following.

Step 1. Work out the mean of the numbers.

Step 2. Subtract the mean average from each of the numbers to gain deviations.

Step 3. Square (times by itself) each of the deviations to get squared deviations.

Step 4. Add together all the squared deviations to get the sum of the squared deviations.

Step 5. Divide the sum of the squared deviations by the number of people in the sample minus 1 to find the variance.

Step 6. Find the square root of the variance to compute the standard deviation.

Example
Step 1. $1 + 3 + 3 + 4 + 4 = 15$, 15 divided by $5 = 3$, mean $= 3$

Score	Mean	Deviation **(Step 2)**	Squared deviation **(Step 3)**
1	3	$1 - 3 = -2$	$2 \times 2 = 4$
3	3	$3 - 3 = 0$	$0 \times 0 = 0$
3	3	$3 - 3 = 0$	$0 \times 0 = 0$
4	3	$4 - 3 = 1$	$1 \times 1 = 1$
4	3	$4 - 3 = 1$	$1 \times 1 = 1$

Step 4. $4 + 0 + 0 + 1 + 1 = 6$

Step 5. 6 divided by $(5 - 1)$, 6 divided by $4 = 1.5$

Step 6. Square root of 1.5 = 1.22. Standard deviation $= 1.22$

This finding suggests that there is less variability in people's visits to the learning disability nurse (standard deviation $= 1.22$) than there is in people's visits in the other ward (standard deviation $= 2.34$).

Statistics

Severity of learning disability

N	Valid	24
	Missing	0
Std. Deviation		27.649

Severity of learning disability

		Frequency	Percentage	Valid percentage	Cumulative percentage
Valid	20	6	25.0	25.0	25.0
	40	6	25.0	25.0	50.0
	80	11	45.8	45.8	95.8
	100	1	4.2	4.2	100.0
	Total	24	100.0	100.0	

Figure 3.13 SPSS output window (standard deviation)

sets of findings, because then you can also compare the dispersion of scores. What is important is that it is good practice always to report the semi-interquartile range when reporting the median average statistic, and to report the standard deviation when reporting the mean average statistic.

Finally, if you do not have access to a computer, we show you how to work out the semi-interquartile range and standard deviation by hand – see Box 3.1.

Making changes to variables

So far in this chapter we have considered describing the properties of single variables. However, what happens if you want to make changes to variables in an SPSS for Windows dataset? Next in this chapter, we are going to show you how researchers change and combine variables to produce new variables. In SPSS these procedures are called *recoding* and *computing*.

● Recoding

There are times when you might want to change the values that have been assigned to particular variables. There are potentially numerous times when you might want to do this: you may have made a mistake typing in your data, you might have changed your mind about how you have coded a variable, you might be working on someone else's dataset and decided to change the coding, you might be dealing with items that are coded in different ways and you want to make them consistent . . . the possibilities are numerous. Changing the values assigned to the data is fairly easy in SPSS for Windows and you can do this in two ways:

- changing scores within the variable;
- changing scores and creating a new variable.

Changing scores within the variable

For this example we are going to use a variable in the adult branch nursing dataset (so you will need to load this up in SPSS for Windows). This dataset has a number of questions asked of 74 individuals relating to a person's physical and general health including their physical functioning, their amount of bodily pain, and their emotional well-being. For our purposes there is one question in the dataset where we have made a little mistake.

We asked respondents how well they were feeling, and they responded on a five-point scale: 1 = Extremely well, 2 = Slightly well, 3 = Neither well nor unwell, 4 = Slightly unwell and 5 = Extremely unwell. We are due to present the findings at a conference, but we decided that since we are trying to measure how well the patients are, it would be better to present higher scores as representing higher levels of being well. There is no statistical reason for doing this but it will just make the presentation of the findings clearer in the minds of the audience, particularly if we are using it alongside other indices of wellness.

Now, we could either recode all the data ourselves or we could let SPSS do it for us. To do this in SPSS click on the **Transform** pull-down menu, click on **Recode**, and then **Into Same Variable** (you will get a Window like that in Figure 3.14a). Then transfer the variable Howwell from the left-hand box into the right-hand box using the arrow button, and then click on **Old and New Values…**. You will now get a Window that looks like that in Figure 3.14(b).

Now you need you tell the computer what values to recode. Here, there are five possible answers to each question. For our question 'How well is the person feeling?' answers scored as 5 need to be recoded as 1; answers scored as 4 need to be recoded as 2; 3 will be recoded as 3, as it is still in the middle; 2 needs to be recoded 4, and 1 needs to be recoded 5. To do this:

- Type **5** in the **Value:** box on the left-hand side (the **Old Value** side), and type **1** in the **Value:** box on the right-hand side. Then press the **Add** button next to the **Old** --> **New:** box.
- Type **4** in the **Value:** box on the left-hand side (the **Old Value** side), and type **2** in the **Value:** box on the right-hand side, and then press the **Add** button next to the **Old** --> **New:** box.

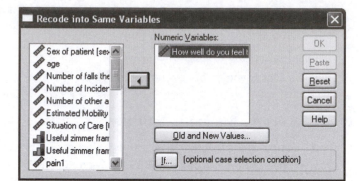

(a)

(b)

Figure 3.14 Recoding the same variable. (a) Recode into Same Variables window. (b) Old and New Values window: upper window, layout in older versions of SPSS for Windows; lower window, layout in newer versions of SPSS for Windows

- Type **3** in the <u>Val</u>ue: box on the left-hand side (the **Old Value** side), and type **3** in the **Val**ue: box on the right-hand side, and then press the **<u>A</u>dd** button next to the **Ol<u>d</u>** --> **New:** box.

- Type **2** in the <u>Val</u>ue: box on the left-hand side (the **Old Value** side), and type **4** in the **Val**ue: box on the right-hand side, and then press the **<u>A</u>dd** button next to the **Ol<u>d</u>** --> **New:** box.

- Type **1** in the <u>Val</u>ue: box on the left-hand side (the **Old Value** side), and type **5** in the **Val**ue: box on the right-hand side, and then press the **<u>A</u>dd** button next to the **Ol<u>d</u>** --> **New:** box.

When you have done this press **Continue**. You will now go back to the Recode into Same Variables window. Press **OK**. The computer will now do recode the variables. Unfortunately you won't be able to see the changes, but it will tell you if there is a problem. So now:

5 = Extremely well (where previously it was 1)

4 = Slightly well (where previously it was 2)

3 = Neither well nor unwell (where previously it was 3)

2 = Slightly unwell (where previously it was 4)

1 = Extremely unwell (where previously it was 5).

You can swap any number you want to. You can turn 5 into 3, 2 into 1, and do it for any numbers you wish. You can be a veritable magician of numbers. However, this method can lead to problems: What happens if you forget you did this? What happens if you make a mistake? Then you might want to explore this option.

Changing scores and creating a new variable

Using the Recode into Different Variables procedure you are able to create a new variable that alters the code given to values but leaves the original variable as it is in the dataset (you may, for example, want to use the original variable with its original codes at a later date). One of the most common examples of recoding like this is when you want to condense the levels of a variable and assign new meaning to the values. Let's try it with our Howwell variable, and let's recode the five levels,

5 = Extremely well

4 = Slightly well

3 = Neither well nor unwell

2 = Slightly unwell

1 = Extremely unwell

into a new three-level variable, comprising those respondents who are well, those who feel neither well nor unwell, and those who feel unwell. Therefore, in terms of recoding the values, we might:

- Recode 5 and 4 into a 'Well' value – making this into a new value of 3.
- Recode 3 into a 'Neither well nor unwell' value – making this into a new value of 2.
- Recode 2 and 1 into an 'Unwell' value – making this into a new value of 1.

To do this in SPSS for Windows, click on the **Transform** pull-down menu, click on **Recode**, and then **Into Different variable**. You will arrive at Recode into Different Variables window (see Figure 3.15a). Transfer **Howwell** to recode from the list of variables on the left-hand side of the Window to the **Numerical Variable** --> **Output Variable:** box. Then you need to give the new variable you wish to create a new name in the **Name** slot in the **Output Variable** box on the right-hand side. Let us call this **Howwell2**. Transfer this new name into the centre **Input Variable** --> **Output Variable:** box by clicking on the **Change** button. To reassign the values, click on the **Old and New Values** and you will go to the same Window as you had for Recode into Same Variable procedure (see Figure 3.15b).

Recode the variable values by placing old values in the left-hand box and new values in the right-hand box. So here we are recoding:

- 5 and 4 as 3
- 3 as 2
- 2 and 1 as 1.

Remember to press **Add** for each recode. When you have finished press **Continue** and then **OK** and SPSS for Windows will compute the new values. You will be able to check you've done this by going to the right of your data, and a new variable, **Howwell2**, should have appeared on your datasheet.

Computing

It is often the case that the variables cannot be measured on just one dimension. There may be several elements within a single variable. Variables such as depression and happiness are made up of many different types of thought and feeling. This is why you see scales in research. Because this has been found to be the case for many variables, researchers, rather than use single variables, tend to use a number of variables together to measure something.

By complete coincidence, we happen to have three such items in the adult dataset. These three items are used in consultation to measure body pain on a particular day among people who have recently experienced some body pain and who have come to be examined. This measure contains three items:

1 The *degree* of pain on that day, with responses ranging from 1 = None at all, to 5 = Extremely painful. This is **pain1** in the dataset.

(a)

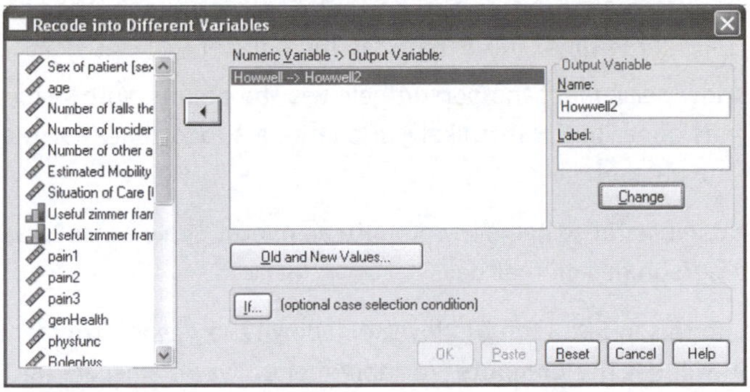

(b)

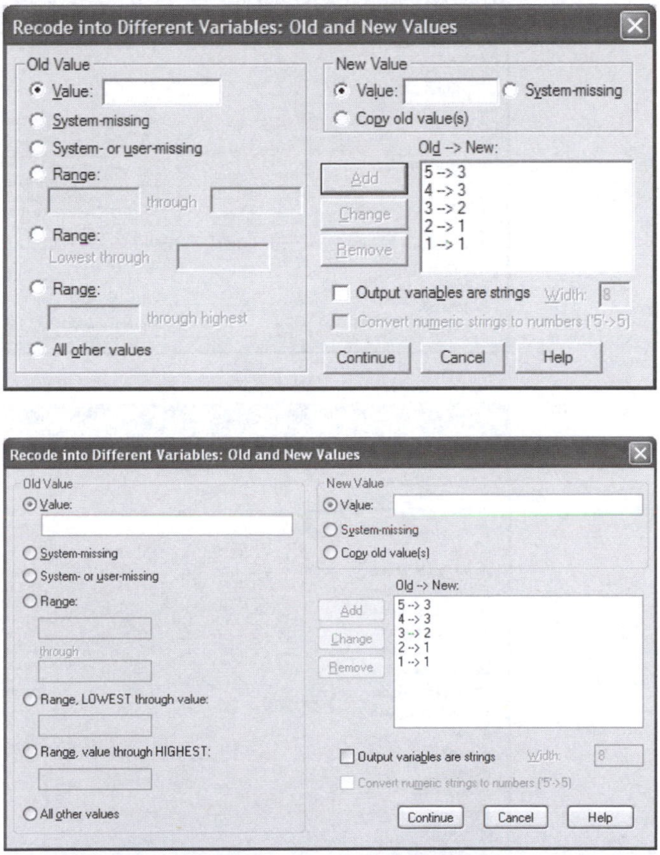

Figure 3.15 *Recoding into different variables. (a) Recode into Different Variables window. (b) Old and New Values window: upper window, layout in older versions of SPSS for Windows; lower window, layout in newer versions of SPSS for Windows*

2 How *constant* the pain is on that day, with responses ranging from 1 = Never, to 5 = All the time. This is **pain2** in the dataset.

3 How *permanent* the person believes the pain is, with responses ranging from 1 = It has gone, to 5 = It is likely to continue a long time into the future. This is **pain3** in the dataset.

We can use these items to compute an overall scale score to assess the amount of pain the person has on that day.

To do this in SPSS for Windows, pull down the **Transform** menu and click on **Compute**. You will get the **Compute Variable** menu. Type Painscale (although this can be called

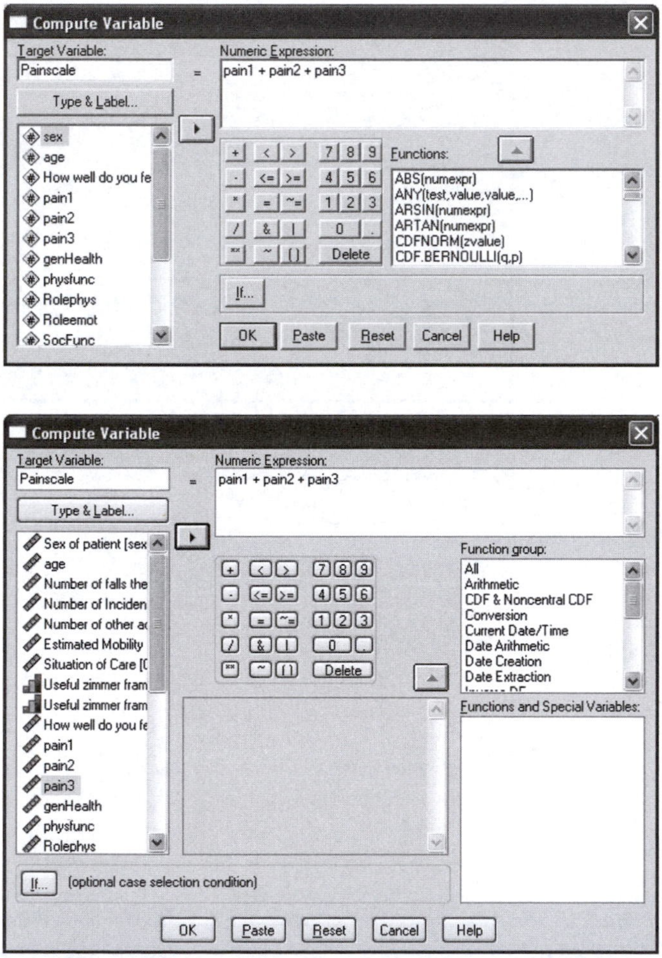

Figure 3.16 Compute Variable window. (a) Layout in older versions of SPSS for Windows. (b) Layout in newer versions of SPSS for Windows

anything you like) into the **Target Variable:** box. Transfer **pain1** from the box on the left into the **Numeric Expression** box. Now click on the + button on the numeric keypad section just below that. Transfer **pain2** from the box on the left into the **Numeric Expression** box and click on the + button on the numeric keypad section just below that. Repeat this for **pain3**, pressing + each time, except after **pain3** (see Figure 3.16).

When you have done that, press **OK**. You will return to the datasheet, and, if you explore along the data, you will see the new variable, Painscale, has been created at the end. You will see that scores range from 3 to 15 on the scale.

We could then assess individuals' daily pain on this scale. If individuals scored near to 15 on the scale then they could be seen as being in a lot of pain that day and perhaps in need of immediate attention. If people responded nearer to 3 on all the answers then they could be assessed as not being in much pain on that day, and perhaps not in so much need of immediate attention, but the report of pain needs further investigation.

Summary

We have introduced you to descriptive statistics, and, more specifically, frequency counts, averages, a measure of dispersion, bar charts and histograms. We have also introduced you to a couple of techniques in statistics that allow you to alter the structure of your data: the Recode and Compute commands.

By now you should be able to:

✔ demonstrate knowledge of frequency counts, averages, a measure of dispersion, bar charts and histograms, and how to obtain these statistics on SPSS for Windows;

✔ perform in SPSS for Windows techniques in statistics that allow you to alter the structure of your data: the Recode and Compute commands.

In the next chapter we are going to introduce you to ways of thinking about and dealing with variables and data.

Self-assessment exercise

In the following exercises we are going to test your knowledge of descriptive statistics by getting you to explore the nursing branch datasets. Select a dataset that is appropriate to your branch of nursing and load it up. For your dataset, answer the corresponding questions. Guidance and answers to these questions are provided on the book's website at **www.pearsoned.co.uk/maltby**.

Adult branch

This dataset contains data on 74 elderly adults. We are going to look at four variables in this dataset for the present exercise:

● Sex of the respondent (**sex**).

● Age of the respondent (**age**).

● The number of falls the person has had that has led to their being admitted to hospital (**numberfalls**).

● The number of incontinence incidents the person has had (**incontinence**).

We are particularly interested in the levels of falling and incontinence among older adults because research has shown that falling and incontinence affect many hospital admissions among older people (Loharuka, 2005).

Use your knowledge of frequencies, averages and measures of variability to answer the following questions.

1 How many men and women are in this dataset (**sex**)? What is the mean age of people in the sample (**age**)? Does this differ from the median and the mode?

2 What are the mean, median and mode averages for the number of falls among the sample (**numberfalls**)? What are the semi-interquartile range and standard deviation for this variable?

3 What are the mean, median and mode averages for the number of public incontinence incidents among the sample (**incontinence**)? What are the semi-interquartile range and standard deviation for this variable?

Mental health branch

This dataset contains data on 40 adults relating to their mental health. We are going to look at four variables in this dataset for the present exercise:

● Sex of the respondent (**sex**).

● Age of the respondent (**age**).

● The average number of hours of sleep each person has reported to have had each night over the past week (**hourssleep**).

● The number of psychological treatment sessions completed by patients (**numbersessions**).

We are interested in the sleep that respondents have had, because poor sleep patterns (insomnia and oversleeping) are indicators of poor mental health (*Nursing Times*, 2005). We are interested in psychological treatment sessions to help us understand what level of treatment each of the people in our sample has had.

Use your knowledge of frequencies, averages and measures of variability to answer the following questions.

1 How many men and women are in this dataset (**sex**)?

2 What is the mean age of people in the sample (**age**)? Does this differ from the median and the mode?

3   What are the mean, median and mode averages for the number of hours of sleep each person has reported to have had each night over the past week (**hourssleep**)? What are the semi-interquartile range and standard deviation for this variable?

4   What are the mean, median and mode averages for the number of psychological treatment sessions completed by patients (**numbersessions**)? What are the semi-interquartile range and standard deviation for this variable?

Learning disabilities branch

This dataset contains data on 24 adults who have learning disabilities. We are going to look at four variables in this dataset for the present exercise:

- Sex of the respondent (**sex**).
- Age of the respondent (**age**).
- Number of consultations the person has had with the learning disability nurse (**consulta**).
- The assessment by the learning disability nurse of the level of nutrition the person has (**nutritional**). Scores on this variable range from 0 (very poor nutrition) to 100 (excellent nutrition), with 50 used as a midpoint (average nutrition)

We are interested in nutrition because studies have shown that people with learning disabilities often suffer from poor nutrition or make poor nutrition choices (Goodman and Keeton, 2005).

Use your knowledge of frequencies, averages and measures of variability to answer the following questions.

1   How many men and women are in this dataset (**sex**)?

2   What is the mean age of people in the sample (**age**)? Does this differ from the median and the mode?

3   What are the mean, median and mode averages for the number of consultations the person has had with the learning disability nurse (**consulta**)? What are the semi-interquartile range and standard deviation for this variable?

4   What are the mean, median and mode averages for the assessment by the learning disability nurse of the level of nutrition the person has (**nutritional**)? What are the semi-interquartile range and standard deviation for this variable?

Child branch

This dataset contains data on 40 mothers who have recently given birth. We are going to look at four variables in this dataset for the present exercise:

- Age of the respondent (**age**).
- Whether the recently born child is the mother's first child (**firstch**).
- The amount of time the mother spent in labour (**timeinlabour**).

● Assessment by the nurse of the percentage amount of energy-dense food in the diet that is eaten by the parents (**energydense**). This is a rating from 0 to 100 per cent. A higher score indicates a greater proportion of energy-dense food.

We are interested in the amount of energy-dense food eaten by the parents, because an increasingly sedentary lifestyle combined with intake of energy-dense food among families is thought to influence the rising incidence and prevalence of childhood obesity (Rugg, 2004).

Use your knowledge of frequencies, averages and measures of variability to answer the following questions.

1   What is the mean age of people in the sample (**age**)? Does this differ from the median and the mode?

2   For how many people in this sample is the newborn child their first child (**firstch**)?

3   What are the mean, median and mode averages for the amount of time the mother spent in labour (**timeinlabour**)? What are the semi-interquartile range and standard deviation for this variable?

4   What are the mean, median and mode averages for the assessment by the nurse of the percentage amount of energy-dense food in the diet that is eaten by the parents (**energydense**)? What are the semi-interquartile range and standard deviation for this variable?

Further reading

If you want to read any of the articles mentioned in the self-assessment exercise, they are all available free online (after registering) at the *Nursing Times* website: www.nursingtimes.net/. The references for the articles are:

Goodman, L. and Keeton, E. (2005) 'Choice in the diet of people with learning difficulties', *Nursing Times*, 101(14): 28–29.

Loharuka, S. (2005) 'Incontinence and falls in older people: is there a link?', *Nursing Times*, 101(47): 52.

Nursing Times (2005) 'Insomnia', 101(39): 25.

Rugg, K. (2004) 'Childhood obesity: its incidence, consequences and prevention', *Nursing Times*, 100(3): 28.

You will be able to access the articles by typing the first author's surname or the title of the paper in the Search box on the website.

Chapter 4

Effective data cleaning and management

Key themes

✔ Data cleaning
✔ Datafile management

Learning outcomes

By the end of this chapter you will be able to:

✔ Explain the concept of validity and why it is important in nursing research
✔ Make the data collected more valid by using proper techniques of data cleaning and management
✔ Use descriptive statistics to look for errors in data entry and coding

Introduction

Imagine . . . That you are a nursing student working on a research project into post-operative pain management among surgical patients. One hundred patients have completed pain rating scales and a battery of other questionnaires. These questionnaires have just been returned to you. This seems like much of the hard work is out of the way – just getting patients to complete questionnaires can be a tough job. One thing that you need to bear in mind is that collecting the data might be hard work, but it is only half the job. Some of the patients have filled in only one or two questions on the questionnaire; other patients appear to have ticked two different pain ratings for the same question. Likewise, when you are doing your research you have to ensure that variables in your dataset are coded correctly and entered into SPSS in a proper fashion. The process of going through your dataset in a rigorous and methodical way to spot errors in coding or data entry is known as data cleaning. You can rest assured that you don't need to take any trips to the laundry or do any long soaking of your questionnaires in the bath. There are less messy ways that we will be recommending to ensure that you're doing a proper job as a nursing researcher. The skills that you have learnt in previous chapters will be vital to managing your data in a methodical way. So far, we have looked at the important aspects of descriptive statistics and now know how to calculate means and frequencies of data. We have also looked at how to manipulate your data with the Transform and Recode/Transform and Compute commands. We revisit these methods in this chapter when learning how to manage data in a 'clean' way.

Validity: what it is and why it is important in nursing research

Validity is an essential component of all research and shows that you are measuring what you want to measure. Sometimes, validity, or lack of it, in a set of measurements or in a method is readily apparent: using a thermometer is not a valid way to measure how depressed someone is, for instance. In other ways, validity, or otherwise, is less easy to spot. If nursing practices are based on data that have been poorly managed and not cleaned, then those practices could in fact be detrimental to patient well-being. Before we look at cleaning your data, it is important to be aware of what it means to collect, analyse and represent your data in a valid way. Validity is crucial to having confidence in the results of a study and in their implications for clinical practice. If you base your nursing practice on research with low levels of validity, it is possible that you are carrying out unsafe practice. This is an essential thing to avoid if you are to meet the requirements under professional bodies such as the United Kingdom's Nursing and Midwifery Council (NMC) to show that you are fit to practise as a nurse.

Different types of validity

There are two main types of validity in nursing research: internal and external validity (Polit and Hungler, 1999). **Internal validity** refers to being able to make an evaluation before and after an intervention. In essence, this is when the independent variable has truly affected the dependent variable (the outcome that you are looking for). For example, you may wish to ensure that your health education intervention (the **independent variable**) has improved a person's levels of activities of living (the **dependent variable**). This test of your health education intervention would be seen as having high internal validity if you can rule out all other variables that might affect someone's activities of living, such as their educational level, their social class or their command of the English language. **External validity** is also essential as it refers to being able to generalise the data you have collected to assume that you will get similar findings in different groups (**population validity**) and a range of healthcare settings and conditions (**ecological validity**). For example, if you found in a trial of a drug to deal with clients' psychotic symptoms that the drug had been successful in minimising symptoms and had few side effects, you would want to know that these results could be replicated with clients anywhere in the world and in any setting: in controlled inpatient units as well as out in community mental health care.

How to make research less valid

There are several ways in which the data you've collected can have poor levels of validity. (Note that we have used the term 'levels'. A piece of nursing research is not solely valid or invalid. Try to think of validity in terms of degrees or levels. Even if there are problems with the validity of some of the nursing research projects that you read about, try not to dismiss the research straight away. Research is something that is often done in stages, and it takes time, patience and application of good research techniques to do it well.) One thing that could affect the internal validity of your research is having participants drop out midway through the project – this is known as mortality (or attrition). This does not mean that the participants actually die (although in some studies, unfortunately, the participants do). Mortality is a big problem, as you can see in the case example in Box 4.1.

Another way of reducing the external validity of your research is to use an insufficiently large sample. The following exercise about sampling error will show you why it is important to have a large sample and that ideally it needs to be randomly selected to avoid bias.

This exercise is based on looking at the scores that people with mild dementia have obtained on a memory test (numbers *above* their heads in Figure 4.1). Scores that are high generally indicate better levels of performance in remembering. In this exercise, you need to do three things. First, add up all of the memory scores that you can see

Box 4.1 Study

'They're dropping like flies'! Case study of research into staff morale

Imagine that you are a research nurse employed to study the impact of an initiative designed to improve staff morale in two palliative care units within two hospitals. One of the units has been chosen as the control group – the group that won't receive any intervention to improve staff morale during the study period. Before the initiative, a sample of staff in both units is selected to fill out a questionnaire to measure their morale. Three months after the initiative, the same staff in both units are again asked to complete the same questionnaire. The problem is that very few staff in the control group have filled out the second questionnaire so it would be difficult to compare the two groups. The table below illustrates the responses for both groups before and after the initiative. It seems as if the percentage of those who have responded in the experimental group has leapt up from 66 per cent to 90 per cent. Does this mean that the initiative has made participants more keen to take part in the study? Can you guess what some possible reasons for the low response rate in the control group might be?

Response and response rate (%) for palliative care staff

Palliative care unit	No. of respondents/No. approached	
	Before initiative	After initiative
Unit A (experimental group)	20/30 (66%)	18/20 (90%)
Unit B (control group)	20/30 (66%)	5/20 (25%)

The concept of attrition relates to the amount of dropout that may occur in a study that requires revisiting participants (such as in a randomised controlled trial). In this case study, the control group had a drop in participation rate from 66 per cent to 25 per cent. It has been recommended that if studies involve a dropout rate of 20 per cent or higher from each stage of the study, then researchers should be particularly wary about drawing definitive conclusions (Polit and Hungler, 1997).

There are several possible reasons for the low response rate in the control group after the initiative. For a start, participants will not have experienced any initiative to boost their morale. They may therefore be reluctant to complete the same questionnaire twice if they see little benefit to themselves. Moreover, those who did respond the second time in this control group may represent a more enthusiastic subgroup within the control group. Overall, it is quite likely, with such a low response rate among the control group after the initiative, that a non-representative sample has taken part. Data from these participants might then need to be treated with some caution.

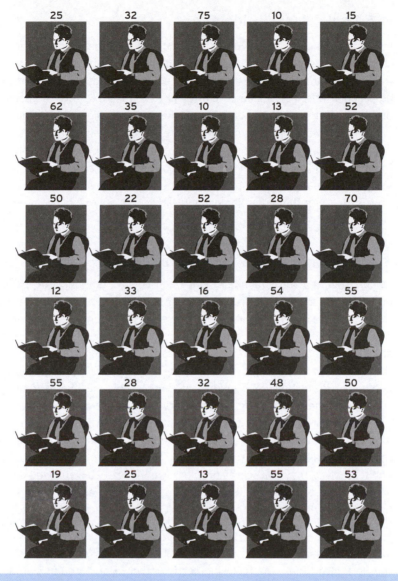

25 32 75 10 15
62 35 10 13 52
50 22 52 28 70
12 33 16 54 55
55 28 32 48 50
19 25 13 55 53

Figure 4.1 *Size matters! The importance of large samples*

associated with each patient and then divide this figure by 30. This score is the mean of the population that you are studying. Second, close your eyes and point your figure randomly at two people pictured in this population. Add up their scores and divide this sum by two. Last, close your eyes and randomly point your finger at ten people and add up their scores. Divide this total by ten. Ask yourself the following questions. Which sample came closest to the population mean that you first calculated? Was it the large sample or the small sample?

Sample size considerations

In this exercise, you chose one small and one large sample of patients. When doing research, we rarely have enough time and money to look at the entire group of people that we are interested in (for example, the population of everyone attending a clinic at a particular hospital). Instead, we often need to take a sample of people and try to get one that represents the population as closely as possible. When you did the exercise above, what was the mean memory score for the small group of patients? And what was the mean score for the large group of patients? Think about what you might have found if you looked at 90 per cent of the population of patients in Figure 4.1. In the small sample you may have got a couple of patients with very high or very low memory scores, but with the larger sample you would probably have got a mean score that is very similar to the population mean.

Sampling error and its impact on clinical care

Let us assume you had limited money and could study only two patients out of the population of 30. What effect will the small sample size have on being able to get a representative group? It is likely that there will be a higher risk of *sampling error* being present. Sampling error is an inevitable part of nursing research where we cannot study the target population as a whole. Say, for example, you chose two patients in the exercise with memory scores of higher than 50 and the population mean for mild dementia was actually 25. In this way, you would be overestimating what people with mild dementia could do on a memory test. This is a big problem because if other clinicians wanted to look at the severity of dementia with the same memory test, they may end up seeing people with mild dementia as having worse memory abilities than the people really possess. What if you had taken a sample of two people with dementia and found that they had scores of 10 or lower. In this way, you would be underestimating the population mean. This poses another problem, as your memory test would not be sufficiently sensitive to be able to tell the difference between someone with mild dementia and someone with moderate levels of dementia symptoms.

There are other ways that your data can be made less valid when you code and enter the data into SPSS. The following section guides you through common errors when carrying out these processes of managing your data.

Common sources of error in data coding and entry

Some of the problems that arise when nurse researchers are dealing with data are outlined in Table 4.1. Just as it is important to work towards tried-and-tested routines when nursing, the whole process of coding your data and entering them needs to be done in a systematic and careful manner.

Table 4.1 Common sources of data coding and entry errors

- Doing data entry and analysis at the same time
- Changing data codes midway through entering the data
- Experiencing fatigue when trying to enter all data in one sitting
- Data coders using different codes to input data
- Not defining values for missing data
- Handling large batches of data at any one time

Simultaneous coding and data entry

As you can see from Table 4.1, errors sometimes crop up when trying to do more than one thing at a time. Entering your data and then doing some data analysis just to see what you're finding will get you briefly out of the routine of what you were doing when entering your data. However, when you go back to entering the data, your brain may be still focused on the creative tasks of data analysis, rather than on ensuring that you enter the data correctly. It is important to take breaks, as fatigue will also lead to errors when entering your data. It is also essential to keep your way of coding the data consistent. If you are coding data with a colleague, you need to ensure that both of you are allocating the same numbers/values to the data you've collected. If you're doing a survey of burnout among healthcare staff and you have the item 'I feel enthused and engaged when at work', are you going to be coding this in the same way as an item such as 'I feel emotionally numb'? It is likely that you and others coding the data will need to sort out systems of reverse coding for some items. (Hint: remember the advice on reverse coding that we gave you in the previous chapter, pages 63–66.)

Inconsistent coding of data

It is vital to have a list of codes that you are going to be using throughout your research. If you are carrying out this study of burnout with mental health nurses and you are coding ward manager as 1 and charge nurse as 2 and later decide to merge the two groups, it is important to ensure that you have used the same codes throughout the process of entering data into this dataset. Perhaps you will want to use Transform and Recode to change these two categories into one, but we urge you to do something like this after entering in all of your data (and not midway through). If you do decide to change some data codes during your research, it is important to make a note of any changes as you progress.

Not dealing with missing data properly and handling datasets that are too large are such common errors when researchers try to manage their data that we devote the next two sections of this chapter to describing how to prevent these errors.

● Handling missing data

When working in SPSS it is important to notice the distinction that SPSS makes between missing data that you define and data that the system notices as being missing. If you leave one of the cells of an SPSS data file empty, then SPSS will label it as missing data. The problem with blank cells is that you need to find out whether these are intentional or whether you forgot to enter data in those cells. Also, if you have taken a file from a spreadsheet such as Microsoft Excel and tried to bring the data into SPSS, it is possible that blanks could be turned into zeros. This could be a problem if scores of 0 are included in variables for which you want to find an average score, as many zeros could reduce the mean score that you eventually get.

Different types of missing data

There are two types of missing data that you need to consider, namely logically inconsistent data and item non-responses. With respect to logically inconsistent data, it would not make sense for a male patient to answer a questionnaire on his experience of being pregnant or of having a cervical smear test. If a male respondent did this, you may need to treat the validity of his answers with some caution. There may also be responses that don't seem to make sense, particularly when you are looking at participants' ratings of how pleasant or acceptable something is. For instance, a patient with psychotic symptoms might say that she prefers the drug olanzapine for controlling these symptoms over the drug risperidone, but that risperidone is better than clozapine. The same patient may then make the seemingly inconsistent assessment that she prefers clozapine to olanzapine. Although this sequential preference of A > B, B > C and C > A may seem strange, we need to bear in mind that people are sometimes logically inconsistent and such responses are still possible. We label these answers from participants as **intransitive response** data, and they should be discounted only with caution. The case of the logically inconsistent pregnant male is a lot more clear-cut and the decision is easier to make when thinking of what data to discard.

Reasons why research participants fail to respond

Item non-responses are another matter. Reasons for these are wide-ranging, such as the respondent forgot to answer, did not know how to answer, simply refused or the question didn't apply to her. If you are able to ask someone why a question hasn't been answered, you may need to build in coding categories to document their reasons, such as 1 = Forgot, 2 = Did not know, and so on. If you are posing questions to someone in a face-to-face interview then it is unlikely that the respondent can forget to answer. However, with postal questionnaires or other means of collecting data where the researcher isn't present, it may be advisable to have a means of approaching respondents at a later date in case some of the items have been missed out through forgetfulness.

Effective ways of dealing with missing data

When you are coding data for which respondents haven't provided any specific reasons for missing responses, it is good practice to document the data as being missing anyway. Try to use a distinctive number that would be unlikely to be a valid response (for example, –9 for a missing response to age). It is also possible that some of the variables in your dataset need to contribute to a total score by summing up several items (think back to the previous chapter when you used Transform and Compute to get a total pain score). If this were the case, then you might want to use the mean score for this item to fill in the gaps for the non-responses. However, you should not treat taking this course of action lightly as, in some respects, you are making up some of your data. It may be likely that the respondent would have given a response close to the mean, but this is still an assumption that you are making for that person. Certainly, if you were finding that a large percentage of your sample had not provided a response to a particular item, it would be foolish to replace the missing values with the mean score that you got for the small percentage of people who actually responded. As we have discussed earlier, you should already be aware of the dangers of increasing sampling error on the basis of having small samples. The same problem applies when using a small sample of responses to generate what *you* think might be the mean score for the entire population of respondents, some of whom did not respond to certain questions.

In the next section, rather than look at errors of omission (that is, missing data) we look at errors of commission (in other words, errors that are actually made by entering the data incorrectly). We guide you through how to spot these errors by using a frequency analysis, the Find command, or other descriptive statistics such as looking at the maximum and minimum data for each variable.

Detecting data entry errors

Using a frequency analysis

There are some simple steps you can take to look for data errors and missing data. What you can do is carry out a frequency analysis for each of your variables. Figure 4.2 shows a typical frequency distribution that you might see in SPSS for a variable called gender. Which areas of potential error can you spot in this table?

Using the Find command

As you will have seen, there were two things that showed possible errors in data coding or entry. The first error was that one person was coded as 3 rather than 1 (for male) or 2 (for female). Why might this be so? It is likely that the wrong key has been pressed by mistake. There is a handy way of finding this error by using the Find command in SPSS. Open the datafile adult branch and follow the instructions in Box 4.2 to find

Gender

		Frequency	Percentage	Valid percentage	Cumulative percentage
Valid	Male	367	88.9	89.1	89.1
	Female	44	10.7	10.7	99.8
	3.00	1	.2	.2	100.0
	Total	412	99.8	100.0	
Missing	System	1	.2		
Total		413	100.0		

Figure 4.2 *Using frequency distributions to detect errors*

the occupational therapist in variable staffmember representing a question on which type of staff member last treated the patient.

With the second possible error in the frequency distribution in Figure 4.2 we found a missing value that has been defined by the SPSS system. This will mean looking down the column for the gender variable on an SPSS Data View sheet and seeing where the blank cell lies. Then you would need to trace the hard copy of the form/questionnaire used where there is an apparent non-response to double-check whether that response really is missing and whether there is any way of getting the data. If there really is no response, we would recommend defining it as missing so that you don't have to search through your forms at a later date. Using the adult branch dataset again, which of the following variables, **numberfalls** (number of falls the person has had), **incontinence** (number of incidents of incontinence) and **nootheracc** (number of other accidents reported apart from falls), have missing data?

Using other descriptive statistics

Another way of looking out for errors in coding or data entry is through carrying out an analysis of the descriptive statistics for the variable in question. In Figure 4.3 you can see that we have generated descriptive statistics for the variable **age**. If, for example, you were an occupational health nurse studying the occupational health status of a group of employees and you got the results shown in Figure 4.3 of the mean, minimum and maximum ages of the employees, would you be satisfied with the accuracy of the data?

	N	Minimum	Maximum	Mean	Std Deviation
Age	406	18	90	27.59	8.60
Valid N (listwise)	406				

Figure 4.3 *Using descriptive statistics to find errors*

Box 4.2 Task

Where is an occupational therapist when I need one? The step-by-step approach to the Find command in SPSS

Step 1. Open the adult branch file in SPSS.

Step 2. You need to look for where the occupational therapist is in your sample. To do so, you should first find which variable can give you this information. To do so, double-click your mouse pointer on the column in your dataset that has the staff group data. This variable has a short label of **laststaffmember** and if you position your mouse pointer over the top of the column you can see the full label for this variable, which is, What type of staff member occupation last treated the patient?

However, for this sample we need you to go to the Variable View screen by clicking once on the **Variable View** tab at the bottom left-hand side of the screen.

Step 3. Now you have a list of variables and information about each one according to variable type, width, the label of the variable and, most importantly, the values used for different categories of response for each variable. This process should be familiar to you after carrying out the exercises in Chapter 2.

Step 4. Now find out what the code for occupational therapist is by clicking on the **Values** button for variable **laststaffmember.** You should see a screen like the one below.

Step 5. You should now see that the code for occupational therapy is 3. This will be what you are searching for. Press the **Cancel** button in the Value Labels window and go back to the Data View window by clicking on the **Data View** tab at the bottom left of the screen.

Step 6. Now click on any cell in the **laststaffmember** column. You have done this to show to SPSS that you are looking for something only in this column.

Step 7. Click the icon on your toolbar that has binoculars on it. This is the **Find** icon and opens a box that lets you search for something in that column. Type in **3** and click **Find Next.** The screen should look like this:

Step 8. As you can see, SPSS has highlighted on row number 57 the data of a patient who was last seen by an occupational therapist. If you wanted to find out whether there was another patient who was last seen by an occupational therapist in your sample, you could click on **Find Next** again. Try it!

Step 9: SPSS has informed you that no further 3s can be found in this column. Click on **OK** and then click on the **Cancel** button in the Find Data in Variable laststaffmember window.

Now, go through a similar process with the same adult.sav datafile and look for someone who hasn't been diagnosed with Parkinson's disease in our sample.

Tips
When you get to the start of step 7, why not try pressing the **Ctrl** button on your keyboard and **F** at the same time? You should get to the same stage. This is handy if for some reason your toolbars get mixed up. Alternatively, try the **Edit** pull-down menu at the top left-hand corner of your screen. Click on **Edit** and you will see **Find** in your list of options. As you can see, there are many ways to get to the same point in your 'journey' using SPSS.

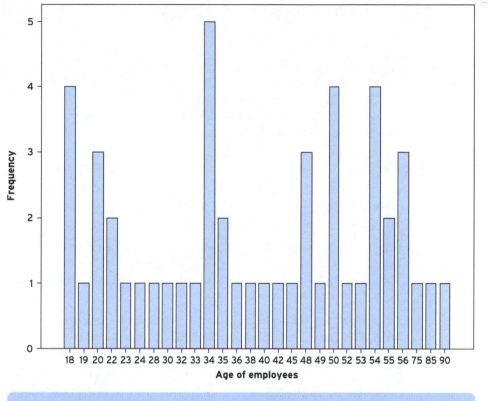

Figure 4.4 *Using a histogram to spot anomalies in data*

As you can see, the minimum age of the employees is 18 years, but there is also a worker who is aged 90. What you would need to do is check with a Find command in the variable **age** to see whether the employee really is 90 years old by then tracking back to the hard copy of their age in their folder in the occupational health office.

Another way to look for possible errors is to use a histogram of how frequently certain responses arise. By looking at Figure 4.4 we can see that there are some employees who appear to be aged over 75. This organisation may allow workers to work beyond the statutory retirement age, but some simple checks with the hard copies of these employees' files may be able to confirm their age status.

● Top ten tips for preventing data errors

To prevent many data coding and entry errors from occurring in the first place, we present in Box 4.3 ten good practices for you to follow. Some of these tips have been adapted from several excellent resources that are concerned with competent data management (Boynton, 2005; Diamantopoulos and Schlegelmilch, 2000; Earnhart, 2003).

Box 4.3 Point to consider

Top ten tips for reducing data coding and entry errors

1. Get someone to read out the data codes to you while you input them into SPSS.

2. Work in pairs to enter the same datasets into two SPSS files. Then compare the accuracy of data entry through frequency tables and histograms.

3. Keep a data diary with a record of your output, the datafiles used, the variables entered and any changes to your coding. This will be a useful way to track your progress and to boost your confidence to look back and see how much you have achieved with managing your data.

4. Do data entry and analysis at different times.

5. Take regular breaks to avoid fatigue.

6. Check your data entered against the hard copies of the forms/questionnaires after inputting each form/questionnaire (or look at a random selection of the hard copies).

7. If only one digit is needed for a variable, restrict the width of the cell. The more digit space, the more risk of pressing a button twice or three times and inputting the wrong data.

8. Sort your 'cases' (i.e. rows of information) to help look for errors. Try to keep the data in the SPSS file arranged in the same order as the hard copy forms of your data. If need be, number each of your questionnaires/hard copies of data and create a variable which allows you to enter this same number for each case.

9. Use value labels for each level of the variable and make the labels informative. In this way you may be able to tell at a glance when a response has been incorrectly entered as all the other cells will be have a label (e.g. with labels such as 'male' and 'female' any number not corresponding with these value labels will stand out like a sore thumb).

10. Save your datafile regularly (every 5 to 10 minutes) and make back-up or duplicate copies. It takes seconds to do and may save you hours of work. You never know when disaster may strike.

● Revisiting good practices for spotting data errors

Try the exercise in Box 4.4.

After entering the data into SPSS, do some preliminary checks by comparing the data you've just entered with the hard copy of the data on the other part of the table in

Box 4.4 Task

Entering data and then checking for errors

The following data are related to the learning disability dataset which concerns 24 individuals who have a learning disability and contains variables on the type of health and ability checks that patients with learning disabilities have had within general practice surgeries. The new data concern the sex and age of the adult who is the main carer for the individual with a learning disability (we anticipate that, over time, a researcher would add data to this file).

Step 1. Open up a new file in SPSS. Label the first column **carerssex** and the second column **carersage**.

Step 2. Enter in the following data for a group of 24 people. Here 1 = Male and 2 = Female for the carer's sex variable.

Carer's sex	Carer's age
1	25
2	33
1	13
2	30
1	35
2	40
1	38
2	38
1	42
2	43
1	56
2	21
1	25
2	65
1	99
2	19
1	39
2	29
1	−9
2	28
2	34
2	55
2	53
2	44

It should look as follows when you have finished:

	Carerssex	carersage	var
1	1.00	25.00	
2	2.00	33.00	
3	1.00	13.00	
4	2.00	30.00	
5	1.00	35.00	
6	2.00	40.00	
7	1.00	38.00	
8	2.00	38.00	
9	1.00	42.00	
10	2.00	43.00	
11	1.00	56.00	
12	2.00	21.00	
13	1.00	25.00	
14	2.00	65.00	
15	1.00	99.00	
16	2.00	19.00	
17	1.00	39.00	
18	2.00	29.00	
19	1.00	-9.00	
20	2.00	28.00	
21	2.00	34.00	
22	2.00	55.00	
23	2.00	53.00	
24	2.00	44.00	
25			

*Untitled1 [DataSet0] - SPSS Data Editor

File Edit View Data Transform Analyze

1 : Carerssex   1

Step 3. What we are going to do with this example is present you with an exercise to get you used to looking for errors in coding and data entry. Now, with 24 people this may not be a problem. However, you may need to ask yourself some questions about the data you've entered. Imagine that you are dealing with a sample much larger than this one (say, $n = 1,000$). You won't have the time or the energy to look for errors in coding and data entry so we will show you in the next few steps how to take a quick route in cleaning your data.

Step 4. Analyse the descriptive statistics. You will be using the skills learnt in the previous chapter. To start, click on the **Analyze** pull-down menu and then click on **Descriptive Statistics** and then **Descriptives** option. Once you have done that, transfer the **carersage** variable into the **Variable(s):** box and click **OK**. You will get an output that looks like this:

Descriptive Statistics

	N	Minimum	Maximum	Mean	Std. Deviation
carersage	24	–9.00	99.00	37.2917	20.29667
Valid N (listwise)	24				

You will see that the minimum age is –9 and the maximum age is 99 years. Something doesn't seem right. You may need to use the skills learnt in this chapter with the Find function in SPSS to locate these anomalies.

Step 5. There may also be other strange entries that do not crop up with the maximum and minimum scores. You can also try another tactic. Before you do so, ensure that you have closed the output window by clicking on the cross on the top right-hand corner of the window. You will be asked whether you want to save this output file. As good practice, it is best to save what you do, so save this output as clean.spo.

(Note: SPSS will usually save this as an output file with an .spo ending. This is to distinguish this output file from a datafile. Next time you want to open it, you need to click on **File** and then **Open** and then **Output** to get a list of the output files you have saved.)

Now you need to look at the distribution of age scores so follow these mouse clicks. Again, click on the **Analyze** pull-down menu and then click on **Descriptive Statistics**. This time you need to click on **Frequencies**. Transfer the **carersage** variable into the **Variable** box. Press **OK**. You will get a table like this:

carersage

		Frequency	Percentage	Valid percentage	Cumulative percentage
Valid	–9.00	1	4.2	4.2	4.2
	13.00	1	4.2	4.2	8.3
	19.00	1	4.2	4.2	12.5
	21.00	1	4.2	4.2	16.7
	25.00	2	8.3	8.3	25.0
	28.00	1	4.2	4.2	29.2
	29.00	1	4.2	4.2	33.3
	30.00	1	4.2	4.2	37.5
	33.00	1	4.2	4.2	41.7
	34.00	1	4.2	4.2	45.8
	35.00	1	4.2	4.2	50.0
	38.00	2	8.3	8.3	58.3
	39.00	1	4.2	4.2	62.5
	40.00	1	4.2	4.2	66.7
	42.00	1	4.2	4.2	70.8
	43.00	1	4.2	4.2	75.0
	44.00	1	4.2	4.2	79.2
	53.00	1	4.2	4.2	83.3
	55.00	1	4.2	4.2	87.5
	56.00	1	4.2	4.2	91.7
	65.00	1	4.2	4.2	95.8
	99.00	1	4.2	4.2	100.0
	Total	24	100.0	100.0	

Step 6. This table presents you with information when trying to find participants who have been misclassified as under 18 years (remember: this is a variable relating to adult carers). You can see that there is a participant who is aged 13 years, one person classified as –9 and another who is apparently 99 years old. Use the skills taught in this chapter to find the case numbers of the people with an age of 13, –9 and 99 years.

Say, for example, you go back and find in hard copies of your data the following:

- The person aged 13 in the datafile is actually 33 – case 3 in the file.
- 99 is missing data – case 15 in the file.
- –9 is missing data – case 19 in the file.

Step 7. Now you have found out what the participants' data should be, you need to recode them or you need to define any missing values. Do it now.

You need to change case 3 carer's age value to 33. And the data for carer's age for cases 15 and 19 need to be recoded as missing. Remember, to recode variables as missing values you need to go to the **Missing** column in the Variable View screen and recode –9 and 99 as missing values.

Box 4.4. Is there anything wrong with the copy you've entered in the file? Before you check the hard copy, do some preliminary checks by looking at the frequency for this variable; look at the mean and maximum and minimum scores for this variable. These values should guide you regarding what to look for. If there are any problems, then clean your data using the principles outlined in this chapter so that your cleaner dataset is in line with the hard copy.

Your final dataset should look like this:

13 is now 33

99 and –9 remain these values but are now coded as missing

Summary

In this chapter, we have outlined:

✔ the concept of validity and its importance in nursing research;

✔ how to make the data collected more valid by using proper techniques of data cleaning and management;

✔ how to use descriptive statistics to look for errors in data entry and coding.

In the following chapter, we will be looking at evaluating the rigour that researchers employ when reporting on descriptive statistics that they have calculated. We will be using a process known as critical appraisal to uncover whether descriptive statistics have been reported in an appropriate and correct way.

Chapter 5

Critical appraisal of analysis and reporting of descriptive statistics

Key themes

- ✔ Critical appraisal
- ✔ Descriptive statistics

Learning outcomes

By the end of this chapter you will be able to:

- ✔ Explain the importance of critical appraisal as a process for evaluating the strengths and limitations of a study
- ✔ Outline a critical appraisal framework for evaluating the use of descriptive statistics in a study
- ✔ Apply your critical appraisal skills by using the critical appraisal framework to evaluate a case study article

Introduction

Imagine . . . That you are a student nurse who has been informed that you and your fellow students need to keep a portfolio to show your professional development and that the portfolio can be inspected by the appropriate body responsible for maintaining professional standards (for example, the Nursing and Midwifery Council). In this portfolio, you need to include information about how well you have progressed on your placements, evidence collected from your placements and information regarding your ability to reflect on your practice. Before you start developing your portfolio, your lecturer has told you that you need to do a critical appraisal of a quantitative study that has measured the pros and cons of student nurses keeping a portfolio. It is up to you to choose what study to appraise and you have come across several, one of which has involved surveying student nurses to find out their experiences of keeping a portfolio. Some of the studies have used rating scales in a questionnaire survey to gauge how a list of advantages and disadvantages related to keeping portfolios applies to each student who responds to the survey. Other studies have entailed getting the students to list the advantages and disadvantages of portfolios and then the researchers have summarised the results by reporting the percentage of students who declared certain aspects of keeping a portfolio to be either an advantage or a disadvantage. There are still several problems you need to resolve. What is this critical appraisal thing that your lecturer has asked you to do, and how might critical appraisal be helpful when looking at how descriptive statistics are reported?

In this chapter you are introduced to what critical appraisal is and how it can be used when assessing the quality of a research study. A system of critical appraisal enables nurses to look at a study in a systematic way and can ease the process of spotting its strengths and limitations. We will use critical appraisal to gauge how well a study has been designed and whether appropriate conclusions have been drawn when researchers have used inferential statistics. When researchers generate descriptive statistics they are attempting to explore their data and to see whether any patterns are arising. The reporting of these descriptive statistics should be done in a clear manner, but sometimes it isn't. By using a critical appraisal framework (a set of questions to ask when assessing the quality of a study), you will be in a strong position to know whether a study has been designed properly and whether descriptive statistics have been correctly reported and interpreted.

What is critical appraisal and why is it important?

Critical appraisal is a process used to evaluate the quality of a study and how it has been reported. This process is often guided by the use of a set of questions relating to study design, how data have been analysed and the conclusions made by researchers on the basis of results. Being able to critically appraise nursing research is a vital skill. Since evidence-based practice became a buzzword for healthcare quality, there has been a growing requirement for nurses to justify using certain healthcare techniques (for example, when could multi-layered dressings be used for patients' leg ulcers and when might they not be appropriate?). Nurses have been encouraged to look critically at their practices and the research evidence to support what they do. This discipline of evidence-based practice is crucial because faulty healthcare delivery based on flawed research could mean the difference between a healthy patient and one whose health is deteriorating.

● Critical appraisal as a way of testing knowledge

A good way to understand the principles of critical appraisal is through the story of the blind men and the elephant (Box 5.1).

The blind men and the elephant

The origins of this fable are unknown, as it dates back many centuries and has been passed from generation to generation and among a variety of cultures. In some stories the number of blind men is three; in others it may be as many as six. It has been popularised in a poem by John Godfrey Saxe (1816–87), who based it in India. The fable goes like this . . .

Many moons ago, in a land far, far away, a group of blind men lived in a monastery away from the hustle and bustle of village life. Every once in a while some of these men needed to go into the village to get provisions and they heard of these beings known as 'elephants', which apparently were useful for carrying people and goods from village to village. Now, being new to these kinds of things, the blind men once made a pact to learn more about this elephant and how they could make use of it. They descended upon the village to have a feel of the elephant and find out what they could do to make use of it. The first of the blind men felt over the elephant's body and cried out, 'My goodness, this beast is very much like a spear!' A few minutes later, and the second blind man had felt elsewhere and retorted, 'You're wrong! It's like a wall. Very sturdy indeed . . .' A third blind man had begun to pull on another part of the elephant as it let out another piercing screech. 'It's none of those, you fools,' this man sneered. 'It's so much like a rope!' And so the explorations carried on, with the blind men coming no nearer to feeling and 'seeing' the whole of the elephant. Each man returned to the monastery still clinging to their 'feelings' and none was any the wiser as to what the elephant really looked like.

Box 5.1 Study

There are several morals to the story, but one of the main ones is to do with the issue of seeing the world from a variety of perspectives. No single blind man was totally correct by insisting that the elephant was like the body part he was touching. However, by systematically using our senses to 'see' the whole of the elephant through detecting the combination of its parts, we can get a better idea of what it looks like. Likewise, by asking systematic questions when looking at a piece of nursing research, we will be in a better position to 'see' the study in a comprehensive way. We will know what the main findings of a study were, whether inferential statistical analyses were appropriately applied and interpreted, what the implications of the results are for nursing practice, and so on.

Critical appraisal as a different way of seeing

Another way of learning more about critical appraisal would be to imagine that you are wearing X-ray spectacles with a range of different-coloured lenses that you could change depending on what you want to look at. By using these X-ray specs when reading about a study, you can clearly see beyond the jargon or statistical tests done to spot any fundamental errors that might have been made. You can also see how the researchers could have designed the study better or how they might have interpreted the data in a different way. If you were wearing the coloured lenses, you could switch from critically evaluating the study's results section in how the descriptive statistics are *presented* (by using blue lenses in the glasses) to examining how the descriptive statistics are *reported* (perhaps with red lenses in the glasses) to how they are *interpreted* (perhaps with green lenses in the glasses).

Critical appraisal as questioning and evaluating

To learn more about critical appraisal, we are going to dissect this phrase and show just how useful this technique can be. Many of you will have used a framework for reflecting on your clinical practice, such as Gibbs' (1988) reflective cycle. With this method, you would be asking a series of questions as you explored the elements of the incident or situation that you were reflecting on. In the same way, critical appraisal is about asking the right questions and coming up with some possible answers. To be critical, you would be looking (with those X-ray specs with coloured lenses) at a study and asking questions such as 'What are the strengths and limitations of this research?', 'Were the appropriate statistical tests conducted?', 'Have the researchers reported the results in an accurate and clear manner?' and 'Is there a justified interpretation of the data and have the authors entertained different interpretations too?' The other part of the critical appraisal concept – doing the appraising (or evaluating) by gathering all your knowledge on appropriate research designs and statistics – is also an essential part of the process. By imagining yourself in the researchers' shoes, you would be trying to evaluate whether the researchers could have done a better job in designing the study, collecting the data, analysing the data collected and interpreting them. In this way, evaluation would consist of making assessments of the components of a study and judging whether it has the overall qualities of good research project. To do this, you would be using a checklist to look at the research in a systematic and consistent way. One thing to note is that just because you spot errors in a study doesn't mean that you should exchange your tinted critical appraisal lenses for black ones that close your mind off to the possibility of the study having any uses whatsoever. It is important to realise that critical appraisal means looking at *how* reliable or valid a study's findings are, rather than seeing the study as either reliable or unreliable. Having results that are highly reliable means that you are likely to find similar results every time, even when different researchers collect the data or different patients take part in the research. Research that comes up with highly valid results is research that is correctly and precisely measuring the phenomen on that the researcher wants to measure. Just as the blind men were not wholly wrong with their perceptions of the elephant, few studies are wholly flawed too.

● Critical appraisal through using frameworks

A critical appraisal framework is a collection of questions, much like a checklist, for you to evaluate how good a study can be. This framework gives systematic guidance on where to look when gauging the rigour of a study. Typically, questions in a critical appraisal framework will cover issues on study design (for example, have the researchers tried to account for bias in getting their sample of patient participants?). It is important to try to remove bias in any nursing study involving the use of statistics. What you want to show is that the researchers haven't had an adverse effect on the outcome of their study by allowing a systematic bias to influence how the participants were chosen. Ideally, in some study designs, it is important for researchers and participants to be 'blind' (that is, unaware) of which participants will be allocated into which study condition so that neither researchers nor participants can inadvertently influence the results. Has there been consideration of extraneous and confounding variables that could ultimately affect the study's results? **Extraneous variables** are variables outside of the participants' sphere of influence (for example, noise or heat in a room), which can have a biasing effect on how participants react in a study. **Confounding variables** are variables that are linked to a participant's characteristics (for example, the extent to which a participant may believe in a certain therapy or treatment).

In this chapter, we are going to be critically appraising descriptive statistics in terms of how they have been used and reported in the Results and Discussion sections of a research report. The whole approach of this chapter entails being logical and following a step-by-step process.

We will be working through a critical appraisal framework to get you to ask questions about the strengths and weaknesses of a case study article that we present to you later in the chapter. Before we introduce the critical appraisal framework, we will show you some problems that sometimes occur when researchers present descriptive statistics. These problems, and more, will be the kinds of thing that you need to look out for when doing the critical appraisal later on.

How not to present descriptive statistics

In Box 5.2 we set out our top ten tips on how not to present descriptive statistics. The tips are a tongue-in-cheek introduction to the habits that would be ideal for creating confusion among the people who read your work. It might be tempting to try some of these tips, but we guarantee that your using them will leave your readers bewildered and unimpressed with the way in which you've presented your findings. Try them and wreak havoc!

Box 5.2 Point to consider

Top ten tips on how *not* to present descriptive statistics

Tip 1. Be plentiful in your use of colour in graphs – very impressive!

SPSS is good for doing colourful graphs. If you don't have a colour printer, then you'll just have to make do with graphs that have shades of grey and hope that the reader can spot which greyish slice represents which label. You need to consider that if you can present your graphs in colour, you may risk alienating the 10 per cent of the male population who find it difficult to distinguish between red and green (Wright and Williams, 2003). Another thing to bear in mind is that many journals do not publish in colour so you will harm your chances of getting published if you send them graphs in colour. However, if you want to really stun your readers, try the 3D option on some graphs. This incorporates all sorts of visual illusions and is guaranteed to blind people with science.

Tip 2. Use graphs with many data points

Look at the bar graph and pie chart below. What is wrong with the pie chart? You guessed it! There are too many bits of data in these graphs. As a rule of thumb, try to have no more than seven categories in a pie chart. If you've got too many categories, it might be best to see if some of these categories can be merged with a Transform and Recode command. For example, some of the categories in the pie chart (for example, birth trauma, congenital abnormality, multiple disabilities at birth) could have been grouped together. You need to bear in mind that graphs are meant to simplify information. When looking at how best to present descriptive statistics in a graphical way, think about what will be clearer to the reader – the pie chart or the bar chart?

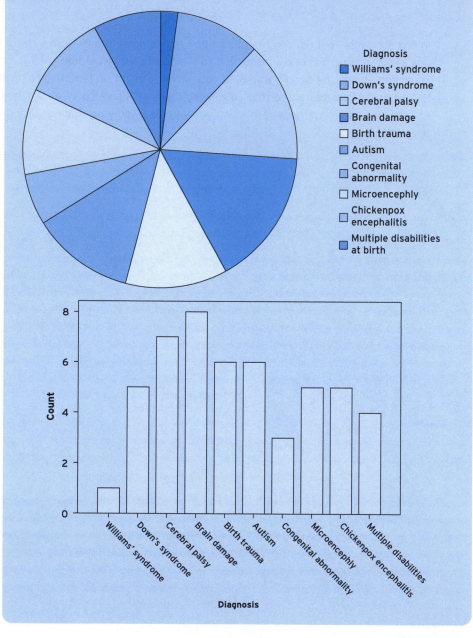

Tip 3. Expect graphs/tables to say it all

One of the most frustrating things to give to a reader is a table or chart that is supposed to say it all. The important thing that you need to bear in mind is that your job is to persuade readers to your point of view. Make sure that you are making a strong case by highlighting the main trends. Don't expect your descriptive statistics to be totally transparent to the readers. Make it plain and simple to them.

Tip 4. Use many graphs/tables when a few words will do

Ask yourself whether that graph/table is really necessary. Is it there to enlighten or just to break up the text like a type of commercial break? Some of the best authors try to avoid overloading their papers with graphs and tables as this may often obscure the message that they want to convey. A sentence or two will do just as well as a fancy graph.

Tip 5. Make it difficult for the reader to see what sample you got and the response rate

A frustrated reader of research papers will often come across an abstract that mentions the sample of prospective participants approached but not the final number of people who actually took part. This is misleading as some readers will initially come across the abstract of a paper and assume that the study involves larger number of participants than it actually does. If you want to mislead the readers even further, avoid giving any response rate as a percentage. Let the readers sort it out for themselves. Here's an example of a particularly misleading excerpt from a Method section describing the characteristics of the participants:

> We randomly selected 275 patients who had used the hospital-at-home service by using a random number generator and the patient lists. We sent them a questionnaire to their homes and 98 completed questionnaires were returned.

With this sort of quote, we have no way of knowing what the percentage response rate was (unless you want to calculate it yourself), we are unaware of how many of the 98 questionnaires were fully completed and how many could be analysed. It is possible that 45 of the 98 returned questionnaires had missing data for over 20 per cent of the questionnaire items. Good practice would involve reporting the percentage of missing data and an outline of how the researchers handled the missing data.

• • •

Tip 6. Report only the means; don't worry about reporting the standard deviations too

The following quote illustrates how thoughtless some people can be. How is the reader able to tell from just the means how the results are distributed?

> The mean pain score for people taking aspirin was 4.5, whereas the mean pain score for people taking the placebo was 5.

A clearer way of describing the results would be as follows:

> The mean pain score for people taking aspirin was 4.5 out of 10 (S.D. = 0.25), whereas the mean pain score for people taking the placebo was 5 out of 10 (S.D. = 4.25).

The results are much clearer and carry more meaning in the above quote regarding the maximum possible score for pain and the closer distribution of pain scores for those taking aspirin versus the more spread-out scores for those taking the placebo.

Tip 7. Inflate the importance of your data by reporting only percentages – especially handy when dealing with small samples

This is a common error, especially in some newspaper articles where there is little mention of sample sizes but plenty of reference to percentages or other ratios in the data (for example, '1 in 5 people preferred . . .'). The following quote sounds pretty impressive:

> Twenty per cent of the patients with leg ulcers preferred low compression bandages for comfort and 30 per cent of the same sample preferred high compression bandages for speed of wound healing.

Compare that quote with a more honest portrayal of the data:

> Four out of 20 patients with leg ulcers who were surveyed expressed a preference for low compression bandages for comfort. Six out of the same sample of 20 patients preferred high compression bandages for speed of wound healing.

Tip 8. Use tables with lots of columns/rows and make sure that the column/row headings are portrayed with a fancy abbreviation

The following table has such a complicated way of measuring with a seven-point response scale that it might be better to merge some of the response categories.

Item	VSA	SA	SomeA	Neither	SomeD	SD	VSD
Able to self-monitor levels	10 (10.1%)	15 (15.2%)	16 (16.2%)	18 (18.2%)	10 (10.1%)	20 (20.2%)	10 (10.1%)
Healthy diet stops my chances of health problems	10 (9.8%)	20 (19.6%)	16 (15.7%)	16 (15.7%)	18 (17.6%)	10 (9.8%)	12 (10%)
Totals	20	35	32	34	28	30	22

Key: VSA = Very strongly agree; SA = Strongly agree; SomeA = Somewhat agree;
Neither = Neither agree nor disagree; SomeD = Somewhat disagree; SD = Strongly disagree;
VSD = Very strongly disagree.

A question to ask is whether the labels for the rows are adequate – what does the item on self-monitoring mean? Is it to do with a diabetic patient monitoring blood glucose levels or is it monitoring levels of well-being for another chronic illness? Another error to commit is not acknowledging whether there are any missing responses to questions. It seems as if fewer people have replied to the first question in the table when compared with the second question. Also, some of the percentages might have been rounded up so the reader may be left wondering why the rows don't add up to 100 per cent. It is good practice to show that you are aware of this issue when reporting descriptive statistics in table form.

What is often very confusing is when authors fail to differentiate one table from another in terms of whether the response scale being used is one where there is more than one response allowed. Here's a table where the authors should have mentioned that more than one option was allowed:

Tutors' perceptions of the disadvantages to students in developing a portfolio

Value	Number of comments
Time required for students and tutors	14
Lack of guidance or clarity in portfolio content or purpose	13
Assessment issues (e.g. not a priority owing to not being assessed)	8
Inconsistent, vague understanding of portfolio concept	8
Low priority	7
Confidentiality and privacy issues	7
Volume of paperwork	3

Tip 9. Use interchangeable terms to mean the same statistical tests/results

Something that is guaranteed to confuse readers is using various terms to mean the same statistical test or result. To do a really good job with this, we recommend that you make liberal use of a thesaurus. After all, the thesaurus is there to make the reader see your work as more interesting and insightful. If you want to mystify your readers, why not do the following?

- Substitute 'mean' for 'average' every now and then. Put in some more words to make it look more sophisticated (for example, words like 'mean average' or 'mean deviation' are pretty meaningless statistically but they look impressive).

- How about using 'deviation' one time and then 'standard deviation' the next? It may even seem as if you've used two ways of describing the distribution of scores rather than just the one.

Tip 10. Use whichever measure of central tendency that best supports your case

There are several measures of central tendency that you could report: the mean, the median and the mode. If you want to make a persuasive case for one group having a better score than another group (for example, comparing a control group of patients and an experimental group of patients who have received a special drug treatment), why not display the *mean* score for the control group of patients and the *mode* for scores with the experimental group? No one will notice if you try to slip in that you're using two different measures of central tendency. It need not matter that you're not comparing like for like. . . . Or maybe you will get caught out.

We hope you have enjoyed reading about some of the definite 'no-nos' for reporting descriptive statistics. Unfortunately, we sometimes find that researchers take up our top ten tips (despite these tips being entirely tongue-in-cheek). Try to make sure that you never commit any of these errors when presenting your descriptive statistics.

A critical appraisal framework to evaluate the use of descriptive statistics

Now you know about some definite 'no-nos' when presenting descriptive statistics, the following framework is a set of questions that have been developed to get you to think critically and to watch out for the mistakes that may be present when authors report their descriptive statistics. In Box 5.3 we cover all the sections that you would typically come across in a journal article, (namely Abstract, Introduction, Method, Results and Discussion). To use this critical appraisal framework, you would need to read through the entire article and evaluate how well the researchers have done. You would be asking these questions as you read the article and would need to add up the number of 'yes' responses at the end. The closer the score is to 29, the better.

Box 5.3 Task

Critical appraisal framework: focusing on descriptive statistics

Circle the answers to the following questions as you read through an article – they are separated according to the typical sections that you would find in a journal article. Add up the number of 'yes' responses. The minimum score that you can get is 0 and the maximum possible score is 29. The closer the score gets to 29, the better the article.

Abstract

1 Are there clear objectives to this study?   Yes / No

2 Was there justification for the selection/generation of the tool
   (e.g. use of validated measure, or development through other
   means such as interviews/clinical audit)?   Yes / No

3 Is the study population clearly defined?   Yes / No

4 Has the method of sampling been shown?   Yes / No

5 Has the size of the sample been mentioned?   Yes / No

6 Has the response rate been covered?   Yes / No

7 Is it readily apparent what the main results are?   Yes / No

8 Are major trends linked to the study's objectives?   Yes / No

Introduction

9 Is there use of descriptive statistics to justify the study's objectives?   Yes / No

10 Is there use of descriptive statistics to justify selection of units of
   measurement (e.g. measuring fluid balance, using kilograms rather
   than grams)?   Yes / No

11 Is there use of descriptive statistics to give a rationale for
   choice of tools (e.g. use of a mercury thermometer or specified
   questionnaire)?   Yes / No

Method

12 Is the population of potential participants mentioned?   Yes / No

13 Have steps been taken to reduce sampling error?   Yes / No

14 Is there an indication of sample size?   Yes / No

15 Was there justification of tools/measures selected (e.g. is there
    mention of validity, reliability or relevance to clinical practice)?   Yes / No

16 Is there a demographic profile of participants (e.g. age, sex)?   Yes / No

17 If 'yes' to question 16, was there a clear presentation of numbers
    and percentages and missing data (if data are missing)?   Yes / No

Results

18 Did the results section start with mention of descriptive statistics?   Yes / No

19 Were there any checks for the reliability/validity of the
    measures used?   Yes / No

20 Were tables clearly presented throughout this section?   Yes / No

21 Was there use of measures of central tendency such as means
    and medians?   Yes / No

22 If 'yes' to question 21, and medians or modes were preferred to
    the mean, was this justified by the author(s)?   Yes / No

23 Were graphs expressed in a clear manner (e.g. were all axes
    labelled, were all pie segments clearly labelled and was it clear
    to which segment of the whole 'pie' each label referred?)?   Yes / No

24 When mentioning percentages in the text, did the author(s) also
    mention the respective numbers for each percentage?   Yes / No

25 Did the author(s) clearly explain the main trends visible in
    the tables and graphs?   Yes / No

26 Did the author(s) refer to a table alongside mentioning the
    main trends?   Yes / No

Discussion

27 Did the section start with the most important findings in summary
    form (i.e. not expressed in the same detail as in the results
    section)?   Yes / No

28 Were numbers and percentages obtained in this study compared
    with figures obtained in previous studies?   Yes / No

29 Were descriptive statistics used to justify the success and
    limitations of the study?   Yes / No

Applying the critical appraisal framework: a case study exercise

As practice in using the critical appraisal framework, you need to now read through the fictionalised article in Box 5.4, which is typical of the kind that you will come across in nursing research journals. When reading the article, you are looking for whether the study authors have answered all of the questions posed in the critical appraisal framework. You will be looking in the Abstract section to find out what the authors think are the most important trends. You will need to look in the Method section to ensure that the method of getting a representative sample is satisfactory and that the authors are using appropriate instruments or materials to collect their data. Most importantly, you will be using the critical appraisal framework to question whether the Results section has presented the descriptive statistics in a clear and understandable way. Do the authors use abbreviations or jargon that is commonly used when portraying descriptive statistics? Do the descriptive statistics show that the authors have fully explored all the possible avenues of enquiry with the data collected? The use of descriptive statistics does not stop with the Results section, as the Discussion section is also one where the authors need to summarise the main trends and show how these patterns in the data either fit with, or conflict with, previous research in the area. Have you found that the authors have done this? Use the critical appraisal framework in Box 5.3 to decide how well the authors have presented the descriptive statistics. Why not try answering these questions now? They should guide your eye so that you look out for the essential components of any article you read. Count up the number of 'yes' responses you get and evaluate how good the article has been in presenting descriptive statistics in a clear and understandable way.

Fictionalised case study article for use with the critical appraisal framework when evaluating how descriptive statistics are reported

Box 5.4 Study

A STUDY OF ORGANISATIONAL AND OCCUPATIONAL STRESS IN A SAMPLE OF NURSING STAFF

G. Willig, G. Sloane and H. Alberts

Abstract

Aims/objectives

To analyse the organisationally and occupationally related stress levels in nurses working in the National Health Service (NHS) of the United Kingdom (UK) according to nurses' levels of seniority

Study

Method

A total of 756 qualified and unqualified nurses were randomly selected from the staff lists of NHS organisations within the north-east of England and were mailed the Nursing Stress Measure (NSM; Goldfish and Bream, 1998), which had been validated with nursing staff samples in the USA and the UK. The NSM measures occupationally related and organisationally related sources of stress among nurses and had been piloted with a group of 25 nurses working within the organisations concerned. A total of 500 nurses returned a completed questionnaire (66 per cent response rate) and 480 useable responses (63 per cent of total sample approached) were analysed.

Results

Greater levels of organisational stress were found among the most senior staff (G grade or above), whereas the lower grades of nurses (C grade or below) had the highest levels of occupationally linked stress. The most salient source of stress for the most junior nurses was dealing with death and dying situations, and those in more middle-ranking jobs (for example, E grade nurses) reported the most stress when dealing with the demands from their managers and subordinates. These findings demonstrate that nurses differ according to their levels of seniority regarding the amounts of stress experienced when facing organisational demands and the daily occupational pressures of the job. This study can be used to highlight the range of staff support programmes and strategies that could be targeted to help the well-being of nurses in relation to their occupational seniority.

Introduction

There have been several major studies of differences within the UK's NHS that have looked at the role of seniority on NHS staff well-being. Two studies, in particular, have analysed over 20,000 staff in each sample (Locke and Plato, 2007; Stephenson and Wright, 2008) and have shown that staff that are lowest in the occupational hierarchy are five times more likely to be absent from work through stress-related physical illnesses and are two times more likely to have psychiatric morbidity than the highest-ranking staff. On the other hand, some studies (for example, Apocryphal *et al.*, 2009) have obtained more equivocal results by showing that high-ranking healthcare staff have a three times greater risk of getting burnout than the lowest-ranking staff. Research among nurses in relation to seniority and stress is less common, although one study by Chill and Blane (2012) has analysed the job stress levels of 64 middle-ranking nurses compared with 23 junior and 15 highly senior nurses. In this study, the authors used the Nursing Stress Measure (NSM; Goldfish and Bream, 1998) to get scores of occupational and organisational stress by using items with a 10-point scale that measured situations that were primarily occupational or organisational in nature.

The authors found that occupationally related sources of stress (i.e. aspects of the everyday part of being a nurse) rated the most highly among the low-ranking nurses. By contrast, the most senior nurses had the highest score in the organisationally related stress component of the questionnaire and the authors attributed this to the intense personal involvement that senior nurses had with organisational issues. The problem with generalising these results to other samples of nurses lies with the small sample that was obtained in this study. As a result, this study was aimed at testing whether similar findings could be obtained in a larger sample of nurses working in several hospitals within the UK's NHS. The Nursing Stress Measure has been chosen to assess stress levels among the nurses in the present study as it has been used in five out of the ten major studies into NHS staff stress over the past decade.

Method

Participants

A total of 756 out of a population of 2,000 nurses working in NHS Trusts within the north-east of England were randomly selected from staff lists obtained from the trusts' respective personnel departments. A total of 500 participants (66 per cent response) returned a completed questionnaire, although only 480 questionnaires had no more than 20 per cent of the questionnaire items missing. As a result, data from only 480 participants was analysed. Thirty-four per cent of the final sample was male and the mean age of the participants was 35.6 years (S.D. = 10.89).

Instruments

The Nursing Stress Measure (NSM; Goldfish and Bream, 1998) is a psychometrically validated tool of 20 items (10 items per scale), which is used to assess two main types of situations that commonly affect nurses: the occupational demands of providing care and the organisational pressures brought about by administrative and supervisory aspects of the nursing role. The NSM has been found to have satisfactory levels of construct validity and the internal consistency of the two scales is also high, with Cronbach's Alpha ranging from 0.90 to 0.95 for occupational stress and Cronbach's Alpha ranging from 0.95 to 0.97 for organisational stress in some studies (for example, Willig and Clow, 2000; Wilberforce and Wright, 2010).

Procedure

Questionnaires and information sheets were attached to the payslips of prospective participants. Participants were asked to complete and return the questionnaire within a period of one week. Completed forms were then to be sent to an address external to their employing organisation. All participants were to give their questionnaire a codename in case they wanted to withdraw their data from consideration at any time within a two-week 'cooling-off' period.

Results

The overall sample's mean scores for the two scales of the NSI are outlined in Table 1, along with the scores for the high-, middle- and low-ranking nurses surveyed. In general, the sample had slightly higher scores for occupational stress when compared with the norm of 50 within the test manual although the organisational stress levels are lower than the norm of 55.

Table 1: Mean scores (and standard deviations) for the NSI - overall and by seniority

	Occupational stress	Organisational stress
Overall ($n = 480$)	58.30 (12.43)	52.50 (10.20)
High-ranking nurses ($n = 200$)	50.23 (12.80)	60.25 (5.30)
Middle-ranking nurses ($n = 180$)	50.50 (19.23)	50.55 (18.12)
Low-ranking nurses ($n = 100$)	65.24 (8.54)	25.40 (5.50)

Note: Maximum possible score is 100 for each scale; the higher the score, the greater the stress.

There was also a supplementary analysis (see Table 2) of the specific sources of stress among the different levels of seniority within the nursing sample. The most prominent source of stress for lower-ranked nurses was that of dealing with death and dying and the demands placed in tending to the needs of patients and relatives during that time. By contrast, high-ranking nurses were most affected by organisational issues relating to conflicts between departments.

Table 2: Mean scores (and standard deviations) for the most and least stressful situation in relation to participant seniority

Seniority	Most stressful situation	Least stressful situation
High-ranking nurses ($n = 200$)	Conflict between departments: $M = 7.20$ (2.50)	Dealing with demands from those lower/higher than me: $M = 2.56$ (5.20)
Middle-ranking nurses ($n = 180$)	Dealing with demands from those lower/higher than me: $M = 6.80$ (2.30)	Periods of inactivity: $M = 2.45$ (5.35)
Low-ranking nurses ($n = 100$)	Dealing with death and dying: $M = 7.25$ (2.53)	Periods of inactivity: $M = 1.39$ (5.24)

Discussion

Main findings

This study has been able to show that stress levels among high-ranking nurses were the highest when it came to dealing with organisationally related sources of stress, whereas low-ranking nurses had higher than normal levels of occupation-related stress, which focused on the demands of dealing with patients, especially with situations dealing with death and dying. It was apparent that middle-ranking nurses did not have stress levels greater than the norm for both occupational and organisational stress, although they did experience a markedly high level of stress when facing demands from both subordinates and their superiors.

Strengths and limitations of the study

The final response rate of 63 per cent was satisfactory and better than previous studies with UK nurses that have had response rates ranging from 25 to 40 per cent. However, it would have been helpful to have looked at the characteristics of the non-respondents and compare them with the participants as we would be keen to avoid over-representing participants who are highly stressed.

Implications of study findings

This study has demonstrated that nurses of differing levels of seniority appear to face sources of stress that are unique to their occupational roles. However, we would recommend exercising caution with the findings, especially as other factors such as personality and internal/external resources available to the individual nurse may have some impact on the ways in which stress is perceived and the ways in which s/he tries to cope. There could be potential for developing targeted interventions to help nurses cope with sources of stress linked to their seniority although this may need to be trialled to see if such efforts are effective in reducing such stress levels.

Summary

In this chapter we have:

- ✔ introduced you to the concept of critical appraisal and explained why it is important in nursing research;

- ✔ examined how descriptive statistics can be used to confuse the reader with our top ten tips on how *not* to present them;

- ✔ outlined a critical appraisal framework to evaluate how clearly you present your own descriptive statistics and how well your nursing colleagues do the same;

- ✔ enabled you to practise your critical appraisal skills by using the framework to evaluate a case study article.

In the past few chapters we have been concentrating on descriptive statistics. In the next chapter, we are going to introduce you to a new set of statistics: inferential statistics.

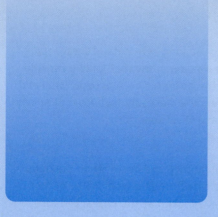

Chapter 6

An introduction to inferential statistics

Key themes

✔ Distributions

✔ Probability

✔ Statistical significance

✔ Parametric and non-parametric statistical tests

✔ Chi-square

Learning outcomes

By the end of this chapter you will be able to:

✔ Outline what is meant by terms such as distribution, probability and statistical significance testing

✔ Outline the importance of probability values in determining statistical significance

✔ Outline the decision-making process about what informs the use of parametric and non-parametric statistical tests

✔ Determine a statistically significant result

✔ Carry out the chi-square statistical test

Introduction

Imagine . . . That you are an infection-control nurse working in a hospital where there is a particular problem with the spread of MRSA (that is, a contact-borne infection that is sometimes found among hospital patients). You have been given the job to promote the adherence to effective infection-control procedures among staff, patients and visitors and have been tasked with reducing the spread of MRSA with the use of various hand-washing methods. In several units within the hospital, you are getting staff to trial an alcohol-based handwash and you want to compare the infection rate in these units versus that in units that don't use such methods. If you find any differences in infection rates between these units, will these differences be down to luck or could they be due to a statistically significant effect? In this and the following chapters you will be introduced to inferential statistics and shown how to make inferences (that is, assumptions) about your research results that will tell you whether your results are due merely to chance or whether they are due to a real statistical effect. We will be returning to the case example of infection control in hospitals later in this chapter.

So far, in this book, we have introduced you to statistics and procedures that have described single variables: frequency tables, mean scores, bar charts. However, the truly magical aspects of statistics are yet to come. One of the main functions of statistics is to explore relationships between variables. Have you ever wondered whether, if you work all your life, you will receive your just rewards? Ever wondered whether the amount of money you invest in improving your house is reflected in its final value? Ever wondered whether level of care administered to patients is really related to remission rates? Well, collect the data, and statistics can be used to provide a definitive answer.

In the next two chapters you will be introduced to a series of inferential statistical tests. This chapter is designed to give you a brief overview of the rationale behind the use of inferential statistical tests. It will not go into a lot of statistical thinking and theory, as we feel this will put you off reading more, and overcomplicate many of the things you need to know. Our main aim is to get you started with statistics, so we are going to give you a simple and straightforward guide to the main ideas. If you want to read more about some of these issues and some advanced thinking, we will expand on these in Chapter 10.

Energiser

Before you start, we are going to get your brain warmed up mathematically and get you to carry out some simple calculations. These calculations are related to some of the concepts you will come across in the chapter.

1. Which is a smaller number, 0.05 or 0.01?
2. Which is the larger number, 0.05 or 0.001?

3. Is the number 0.10 larger or smaller than 0.05?

4. Is the number 0.50 larger or smaller than 0.01?

5. Between which two numbers does 0.02 fit in this series?

      0.50   0.30   0.10   0.05   0.01

6. Between which two numbers does 0.20 fit in this series?

      0.50   0.30   0.10   0.05   0.01

Distributions

In Chapter 3 you were shown how to create a histogram on SPSS for Windows (the distribution of scores for a continuous-type variable). Researchers have identified different types of distribution of a histogram to introduce an idea that is a cornerstone of statistics. This idea is based on different ways of describing distributions.

Histograms can be described as *skewed* (see Figure 6.1), either negatively (where scores are concentrated to the right) or positively (where scores are concentrated to the left). An example of a distribution of a **negatively skewed distribution** may occur when high scores on the variable are highly desirable. Therefore, if researchers develop a 'kindness' scale (in which higher scores indicate a higher level of kindness) containing

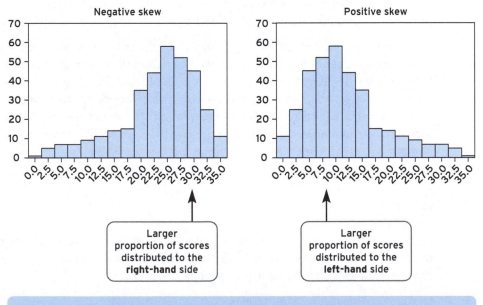

Figure 6.1 Negatively and positively skewed distributions

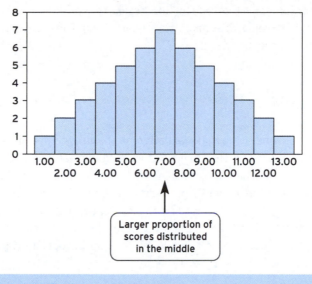

Larger proportion of
scores distributed
in the middle

Figure 6.2 *Normal distribution*

items such as 'I am kind to other people' and 'I am a very kind person', we might expect most respondents to view themselves as being kind, as opposed to being unkind. Therefore, a negative skew would emerge as people respond with high 'kindness' scores. An example of a **positively skewed distribution** of a variable is often found with measures of depression. Measures of depression tend to identify greater and greater degrees of severity of depression, so researchers often find that most respondents score low on depression, as most people are not regularly depressed, and few people have high scores (as the highest scores indicate severe depression, and few respondents tend to be clinically depressed).

The final description is where the distribution of scores for a variable forms a **normal distribution**. This is where scores are distributed symmetrically in a curve, with the majority of scores in the centre, then spreading out, showing increasingly lower frequency of scores for the higher and lower values (Figure 6.2).

What is particularly notable about this is that researchers have found that many variables measuring human attitudes and behaviour follow a normal distribution. This finding is one of statistics' more interesting elements. Statisticians and researchers are often not certain why many variables fall into a normal distribution; they have simply found that many attitudes and behaviours do so.

However, statisticians have noted that if scores on a variable show a normal distribution, then they have a potentially powerful statistical tool. This is because we can then begin to be certain about how scores will be distributed for any variable; that is, we can expect many people's scores to be concentrated in the middle and few to be concentrated at either end of the scale. This certainty has given statisticians the impetus to develop ideas about statistical testing. These developing ideas centre on the concept of probability.

Probability

With the advent of the National Lottery in the UK, the use of the word 'probability' has increased in society. The chances of winning the National Lottery jackpot are thought to be about 14 million to 1, meaning that there is a very small probability that you will win. We can make a number of assertions about life based on probability. It is 100 per cent probable, if you are reading this sentence, that you have been born; there is a 50 per cent probability (1 in 2) that a tossed coin will turn up heads (50 per cent probability that it will turn up tails), 16.66 per cent probability (1 in 6) that a roll of a die will show a 6.

Some of the ideas about uses of probability in statistics have come from recognising that scores are often normally distributed. With normal distribution we are able to talk about how individual scores might be distributed. An example of this would be for a variable in which scores are normally distributed between 0 and 10. We would then expect most scores (the most probable) to be around 5, slightly fewer scores around 6 and 4, slightly fewer scores again around 7 and 3, and so on (8 and 2; 9 and 1), until the least expected scores (the least probable) are 0 and 10.

These expectations lead us to the key issue emerging from probability: the idea of confidence. Researchers use probability to establish confidence in their findings. The reason why researchers are concerned with establishing confidence in their findings is a consequence of their using data that are collected from **samples**. Owing to constraints of time, money or accessibility to possible respondents, researchers always use sample data to generalise, or make **statistical inferences** (hence the generic name of *inferential* statistics for the tests we will use in the next few chapters), about a **population**. This means that there is always a chance that researchers will make an error, because they never have access to the whole population, and therefore can never be certain of how every possible respondent would have scored on a variable. However, because researchers find that variables often form a normal distribution, they can use samples to generalise about populations with confidence. Researchers try to establish confidence by talking about their findings with regard to probability. An example of how they do this can be seen in the horse racing form card in Table 6.1.

At the bottom of this form is the betting forecast. As you can see, Long-term Care is the favourite, at evens, with Call Bell being least favourite, at 33/1. In a similar way to that in which bookmakers suggest that it is probable that Long-term Care will win, and that Call Bell will probably not win, researchers use probability to grade findings as

Table 6.1 Racing form card for the Fantasy Horse Novices' Hurdle

3.40
Fantasy Horse Novices' Hurdle (Class D) (4 y.o.+)   2 m 7$\frac{1}{2}$ fl
11 run   Winner £2,260   **Going: Good**

No.	Horse	Wgt	Jockey
1	Long-term Care	10-12	C. Barton
2	Physical Assessment	10-12	L.M. Alcott
3	Antibiotic	10-12	E. Church
4	Case Management	10-12	E. Cavell
5	Gastrointestinal	10-14	D.L. Dix
6	Foley Catheter	10-12	M.E. Mahoney
7	Cardiovascular Boy	10-12	E. Robson
8	Perioperative	10-12	J. Delano
9	Conscious Sedation	10-12	E. Kelly
10	Tracheostomy	10-12	M.E. Zakrzewska
11	Call Bell	10-7	F. Nightingale

Betting forecast: Evens, Long-term Care; 2/1 Physical Assessment; 7/2 Antibiotic; 6/1 Case Management; 10/1 Gastrointestinal; 14/1 Foley Catheter; 16/1 Cardiovascular Boy; 18/1 Perioperative; 16/1 Conscious Sedation; 25/1 Tracheostomy; 33/1 Call Bell.

more or less probable. However, unlike bookmakers, researchers use criteria to decide whether something is probable or not probable. The way this is done is through significance testing.

Significance testing

Significance testing is a criterion, based on probability, that researchers use to decide whether two variables are related. Remember, because researchers always use samples, and because of the possible error, significance testing is used to decide whether the relationships observed are real.

Researchers are then able to use a criterion (significance testing) to decide where their findings are probable (confident of their findings) or not probable (not confident of their findings). This criterion is expressed in terms of percentages and their relationship to probability values. If we accept that we can never be 100 per cent sure of our findings, we have to set a criterion of how certain we want to be of our findings. Traditionally, two criteria are used. The first is that we are 95 per cent confident of our findings; the second is that we are 99 per cent confident of our findings. This is often expressed in another way. Rather, there is only 5 per cent (95 per cent confidence) or 1 per cent (99 per cent confidence) probability that we have made an error. In terms of significance testing these two criteria are often termed as the 0.05 (5 per cent) and 0.01 (1 per cent) significance levels.

In the next few chapters you will be using tests to determine whether there is a **statistically significant** association or relationship between two variables. These tests always provide a probability statistic in the form of a value, for example 0.75, 0.40, 0.15, 0.04, 0.03, 0.002. Here, the notion of significance testing is essential. This probability statistic is compared against the criteria of 0.05 and 0.01 to decide whether our findings are statistically significant. If the **probability value** (p) is less than 0.05 ($p < 0.05$) or less than 0.01 ($p < 0.01$) then we conclude that the finding is statistically significant.[1] If the probability value is more than 0.05 ($p > 0.05$) then we conclude that our finding is not statistically significant. Therefore, we can use this information in relation to our research idea and we can determine whether our variables are statistically significantly related. To summarise for the probability value stated above:

- The probability values of 0.75, 0.40 and 0.15 are greater than 0.05 (> 0.05) and these probability values are not statistically significant at the 0.05 level ($p > 0.05$).

- The probability values of 0.04 and 0.03 are less than 0.05 (< 0.05) but not less than 0.01, so these probability values are statistically significant at the 0.05 level ($p < 0.05$).

- The probability value of 0.002 is less than 0.01 (< 0.01); therefore this probability value is statistically significant at the 0.01 level ($p < 0.01$).

An analogy of significance testing to research is the use of expert witness with evidence in court cases. In a court case, an expert witness is asked to comment on a piece of evidence to help the jury draw a conclusion about the accused. In the same way, the researcher uses significance testing (the expert witness) to help to determine whether the finding (evidence) is significant (the jury conclusion).

Exercise: Using probability and statistical significance

Using the following probability values, decide whether the statistic is statistically significant or not statistically significant. Then decide, if the result is statistically significant, which level of significance the statistic is at (0.05 or 0.01).

1 0.060

2 0.030

3 0.500

4 0.002

5 0.978

So, we now know we can do amazing things with numbers. They are not just numbers: things happen with them. The normal distribution allows us to make statements about

---

[1] Note that if the probability statistic is below 0.01 (say, 0.002) then we don't need to bother mentioning that it is below 0.05 as well – we already have greater (99 per cent) confidence in our finding.

where scores are likely to happen in a population. Probability introduces us to ideas of things being likely to happen or not happen. What these ideas in statistics do is lead us to the idea of inferential statistical tests.

Inferential statistical tests

We are now on to the really exciting stuff. Whereas descriptive statistics were exciting in their own right with their ability to describe single variables, **inferential statistics** can be used to provide answers to our naturally inquisitive minds. As a nurse you are always asking investigatory questions:

- Does the use of this drug make people better?
- Does the length of waiting lists have an effect on patients' health?
- Does medication help psychotic patients?
- Are the attitudes of parents to the MMR jab related to their inexperience with children?

Inferential statistical tests (so called because they make inferences from data collected from a sample to the general population) are statistical tests that take data and provide answers to questions such as these – in fact any question you wish to devise. The only things you need in order to start using inferential statistics are two variables and some data collected relating to those two variables. After that, the statistical world is your oyster.

However, our first problem is that there are many statistical tests. We cover seven in this book. Over the course of this and the next two chapters you will be introduced to each of these tests. Why so many? This is because of two things. The type of statistical test being used depends on:

- the types of variable being used, in other words whether they are categorical-type or continuous-type – we've covered this, particularly in Chapter 2;
- if they are continuous-type variables, whether they should be used in parametric or non-parametric statistical tests.

The latter distinction – parametric and non-parametric – you haven't come across before so we will now explain it.

The importance of the parametric and non-parametric distinction

What do we mean by parametric and non-parametric? Remember that earlier in this chapter we said that if data form a normal distribution then they are very powerful because they allow us to be *certain* about how scores will be distributed in a variable. This certainty then led to the development of a number of statistical tests that allowed us to be confident in looking at relationships between variables. These tests were called **parametric statistical tests**, based on the normal distribution curve.

However, statisticians, in their wisdom, wondered what would happen if we had data that didn't form a normal distribution. Rather than give up and go home, they also developed a series of tests that were to be used when the data did not form a normal distribution and, therefore, were less certain about how scores were distributed within a variable (an alternative, a back-up, a plan B for us all to use). These tests became known as **non-parametric statistical tests**.

So, within statistics, a major distinction is drawn between parametric tests and non-parametric tests. We will go through these in the next two chapters, but an important idea you must get the hang of here is that, with continuous-type data, the researcher must always decide whether the test used to verify them should be a parametric or non-parametric statistical test. The central criterion to help them decide on the type of test is whether or not the data form a normal distribution. If their continuous-type data form a normal distribution, then they should be used in a parametric statistical test; if they do not form a normal distribution, then they should be used in a non-parametric statistical test.

The next question is, how do you tell whether your continuous-type data are parametric or non-parametric? There are two ways to do this. The first is to create a histogram of the data and see whether they form a normal distribution. The second is to see whether your data are skewed, that is, do not form a normal distribution. You can do this by getting a skew statistic on SPSS for Windows. Often it is difficult to tell from a histogram whether the data are skewed. Therefore, you can use the skewness statistic in SPSS to gain an idea.

Let us use an example from the child branch dataset. Load up the dataset into SPSS for Windows. This is the dataset that includes information on 40 mothers and attitudes to factors surrounding their children. In this chapter we are going to look at variables among this sample:

- age of the mothers (**age**);
- the amount of time in hours the mother spent in labour (**timeinlabour**).

Let us first produce histograms for both these variables (this is the same as in Chapter 3). Go to **Graphs** and select **Histogram…**. Then move the variable **age** into the **Variable** box, click the box next to **Display Normal Distribution curve** and press **OK**. You should get an output like that in Figure 6.3. Repeat this with the **timeinlabour** variable and you should get the output like that shown in Figure 6.4.

You can see from both graphs that the distribution of scores can be *compared* against the black line, which is a normal distribution curve. You can see that the amount of time spent in labour forms a normal distribution, but the age variable seems to be skewed towards the lower end (positively skewed). This is perhaps not surprising given that mothers will tend to have babies earlier rather than later in life.

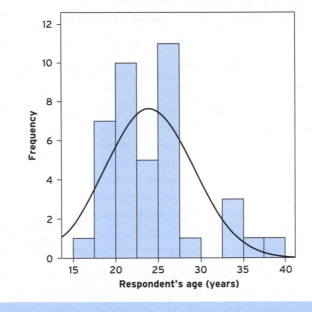

Figure 6.3 Histogram of respondents' ages

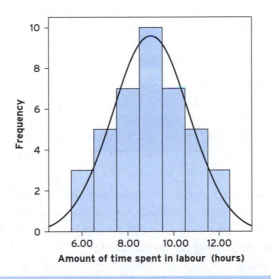

Figure 6.4 Histogram of respondents' time spent in labour

Descriptive Statistics

	N	Minimum	Maximum	Mean	Std.	Skewness	
	Statistic	Statistic	Statistic	Statistic	Statistic	Statistic	Std. Error
Respondent's age	40	17	40	24.00	5.228	1.180	.374
Amount of time spent in labour	40	6.00	12.00	9.0000	1.66410	.000	.374
Valid N (listwise)	40						

Skewness statistic

Figure 6.5 *Descriptive statistics with skewness statistic of respondent's age and time spent in labour*

However, you may see that there are problems with making this judgement. More often than not it is not easy to tell whether a variable is normally distributed. For example, the time in labour variable does seems to have properties of a normal distribution: it has a high middle, among other things. However, it is not always easy to tell whether your data form a normal distribution. Therefore, the other way to approach the problem is to find out whether your data are skewed statistically. You get the skewness statistic. You can do this now from the **Analyze** pull-down menu, click on **Descriptive Statistics**, and then on **Descriptives**. Transfer the variables **age** and the **timeinlabour** into the box, click on the **Options** button and tick the box next to **Skewness**. By pressing **Continue** and then **OK**, you will get the skewness statistic with your output (see Figure 6.5).

The skewness statistic will be either positive or negative, indicating in which direction the skewness may lie. There is a test to decide whether your skewness statistic means you have a skewed distribution, but this is vulnerable to the number of people you have in your sample. Most researchers use a general criterion that any statistic above 1.00 (either + or −) means your distribution is skewed. As you can see, age is skewed but the time spent in labour is not skewed.

Therefore we suggest that the main guideline to use when deciding whether your continuous-type data are suitable for parametric or non-parametric tests is whether the data are skewed. If they are not skewed, then they probably are suitable for use in parametric tests. If they are skewed, then you might wish to use them in non-parametric tests instead.

● The complication with the parametric and non-parametric distinction

So far, the criterion to decide whether data should be treated as parametric or non-parametric seems simple. Do the data form a normal distribution or not? Unfortunately, it is not always that simple in practice. Before we say why, it is as well to know that the question of what constitutes parametric is one that is hotly debated in statistical teaching. Your lecturers may look as if they are all friendly with each other, but if there is one thing that is guaranteed to split a staff group into factions it is their views on the parametric versus non-parametric question. Intrigued? Read on.

You see, there are other rules, and the degree to which they apply, and the importance attached to these rules, vary among statisticians.

Many people have different views about the criteria for deciding whether continuous-type data should be treated as parametric or non-parametric. Our consideration of the different views, debates and split in academic departments begins with three rules, which are generally agreed to be important. The rules of whether continuous-type data should be treated as suitable for parametric test are:

- **Rule 1**. Data should be normally distributed (as already discussed).

- **Rule 2**. The scores on any continuous-type data must be interval or ratio data (or continuous if you are using the categorical/discrete/continuous distinctions between variables). We covered this in Chapter 3; interval or ratio data are variables that are numerical, meaning that they comprise numerical values (for example, age, hours spent in labour), where the actual number means something. This means that the levels of these variables are real numbers that mean something numerically. Therefore, data such as ordinal data, which are of a continuous type but represented by artificial numbers, do not count. For example, a measure of pain where no pain is scored as 0, mild pain is scored as 1, moderate pain is scored as 2, and extremely severe pain is scored as 3 is not a variable of real numbers; instead it comprises numbers we've assigned to understand the amount of pain.

- **Rule 3**. If two continuous-type variables are being used or compared, they must have similar standard deviations. We covered standard deviation in Chapter 4. The standard deviation provides the researcher with an indicator of how scores for variables are spread around the mean average (this is why it is sometimes referred to as a measure of dispersion). The higher the standard deviation, the more the scores are spread out (the scores 0, 1, 2, 2, 0 will have a low standard deviation, whereas the scores, 0, 50, 100, 200, 500 will have a much higher standard deviation).

These are all rules for determining whether your data are parametric. They can be used to determine whether your data are suitable for use in a parametric statistical test.

Furthermore, if your continuous-type data do *not* follow these rules, you do *not* use a parametric statistical test; instead you use a non-parametric test. So, for Rule 2, if your data are not interval or ratio data, then you should use a non-parametric test. For example, consider an ordinal variable which asks the respondent how their anxiety might be scored: 1 = Not at all, 2 = Sometimes, 3 = Often, 4 = Always. It is sometimes argued that this scoring does not reflect numerical properties, as the score of 4, for instance, given for responding 'Always' to the question, does not represent a behaviour that is twice as much as the score of 2, given for 'Sometimes' ('Always' is not twice as much as 'Sometimes'). Similar principles apply for Rules 1 and 3. If your continuous-type data are *not* normally distributed (Rule 1) or if two sets of continuous-type scores are being used or compared and they do *not* have similar standard deviations (Rule 3) then a non-parametric test should be used.

BUT, and this is a big but, people don't always use these three rules. Or, they will vary in the application of these rules. Even when the data do not comply with the rules, researchers may treat data as parametric that look more suited to being treated as non-parametric. They may do this for a number of good reasons, including the following:

- The statistics test has been previously used by other researchers to look at the same variable. This is sometimes done to provide consistency in the research literature.
- Although some continuous-type variables may not comprise real numbers (such as ordinal data which ranks the data), we can make the assumption that they *are* real numbers because researchers are assigning these values to responses.
- Sometimes, researchers will assume their continuous-type data are normally distributed because they have collected data with adequate sampling techniques and, therefore, have data that are in general representative of a variable which would be expected to be normally distributed in a larger population. For example, if you do a study of 40 people then the data will not likely form a normal distribution because you haven't got enough cases.
- The scale used to measure the continuous-type variable is a well-established, reliable and valid measure of that variable and has been shown by previous research (among larger samples) to demonstrate a normal distribution of scores.
- Because their lecturer/teacher has told them so. Lecturers and teachers may suggest you use a certain version of the test because of wider learning reasons or for reasons of being consistent with the literature.

What you need to be aware of most is that researchers do vary in practice and people do not always agree with each other's approaches. People will be very definite about their way of doing things and insist that their way is correct. This is often a source of confusion for students of statistics, and the best strategy you can employ is just to be aware that researchers do vary in practice. Usually, there is little point in adopting one position only, because often you will work with colleagues, complete reports for employers/teachers/lecturers, or submit papers to academic journals that will insist you adopt a different tactic. Ideally, you should be aware that different valid practices exist and be able to employ and engage with these different practices when needed.

It is best to use these various rules and practices as guidelines to decide whether to use parametric or non-parametric versions of tests. However, overall, you should remember that this decision shouldn't be viewed as a big problem. The purpose is not that you should develop a concept of parametric versus non-parametric tests. Rather, you should appreciate that statisticians have provided us with different ways of solving problems. Therefore, there is nothing to worry about if you find that the continuous-type variables you have measured do not show parametric properties: you simply use non-parametric tests as an alternative.

What we suggest you do at this stage, to keep things as simple as possible, is to use the normal distribution criterion and the skewness statistics as ways of determining the parametric versus non-parametric question when it is needed. Then, as you become more experienced with statistics (or as you come across them), you could begin to consider the other rules.

Moving forward

In moving forward to the next stage, you need to remember two things before being introduced to the world of statistical tests, namely that:

- variables can be generally defined as two types: categorical-type or continuous-type (we have covered this throughout the book so far);
- when using continuous-type variables, a distinction is made between whether the data should be used in parametric or non-parametric statistical tests, and this choice rests on whether your data form a normal distribution (we have covered this in this chapter).

Statistical tests and the decision-making table

Let us introduce you to all the statistical tests you will use in the book and the context for using these tests. Remember, the aim of any inferential statistical test is to answer your question of whether there is something happening between two variables. Although there are a number of statistical tests, you use only one statistical test with any one question. *The problem is that you have to use the right one*. How do you ensure you use the right one? Let us introduce you to our decision-making chart (Figure 6.6).

In our decision-making chart you will notice a number of darkly shaded blocks with terms such as chi-square, Pearson, Spearman, paired-samples *t*-test, Wilcoxon sign-ranks test (to name just a few) written in them. These are the seven tests that we will cover in the book and are the end points of the decision-making process.

The aim of the decision-making process is to reach one of these end points. To reach each point, what you must do is to answer *two* questions in each of the columns in turn, choosing your response from the rows below. What you must then do is continue along each row until you reach an end point. Then, when you reach this end point, you should know which type of statistical test you should use.

Question 1 What combination of variables do you have?	Which statistical test to use	Question 2 Should your continuous-type data be used with parametric tests or with non-parametric tests?	Which statistical test to use
Two categorical-type variables	Chi-square		
Two separate/ independent continuous-type variables	Go to question 2	Parametric Non-parametric	Pearson correlation Spearman correlation
Two continuous-type variables, which is the same variable administered twice	Go to question 2	Parametric Non-parametric	Paired-samples *t*-test Wilcoxon sign-ranks
One categorical-type and one continuous-type variable	Go to question 2	Parametric Non-parametric	Independent-samples *t*-test Mann-Whitney *U* test

Figure 6.6 *Decision-making table for choosing statistical tests*

The two questions are:

- What types of variable are being used and in what combination?
- Should the continuous-type variables be used in parametric or non-parametric statistical tests (remember, your answer to this question rests on whether your data form a normal distribution)?

If you are able to answer both of these questions successfully then you will always choose the right statistical test.

To illustrate this process let us use an example. Hospital staff are interested in examining recent findings that women who have an epidural to ease the pain of childbirth are more likely to need medical help to have their baby (see http://news.bbc.co.uk/1/hi/health/4371552.stm). One important aspect to this study is that women opting for an epidural were more likely to experience a longer second stage of labour. Our staff want to see whether this is occurring in their hospital. The researchers have decided to measure the following variables:

- whether or not the mother has had an epidural during childbirth (forming a two-level categorical-type variable);

- the length of the second stage of labour. The staff have found that the continuous-type variable has a normal distribution.

In terms of moving forward, we have to choose which statistical test to use. In answer to the two questions in our decision-making table:

- we have one categorical-type variable and one continuous-type variable;

- the continuous-type variable has a normal distribution, and therefore it is suitable for use in a parametric test.

Therefore, we would choose an independent-samples *t*-test.

Now, we know you have no idea what an independent-samples *t*-test does, but you can see that you can already find your way through different statistical tests. And that skill is an important aspect of statistics. Have a go yourself in the next section.

Self-assessment exercise: Choosing an inferential statistical test

Following efforts by NHS Lothian to combat the MRSA hospital superbug via information packs, leaflets and posters (http://news.bbc.co.uk/1/hi/scotland/4370730.stm), your local health authority has decided to see whether hospitals under its control could benefit from such a drive. Research staff at the local health authority have then surveyed each of the authority's hospitals on two issues:

- whether there have been any special initiatives within the hospital, such as information packs on infection control and prevention given to staff, or posters and leaflets aimed at patients and visitors to raise awareness of the problem. Responses are either yes or no;

- whether the hospital has been given a clean bill of health in terms of there not being a reported case of the MRSA superbug in the hospital. Responses are either yes or no.

To help you, the research staff have decided that both variables are categorical-type data.

What statistical test should the researcher use?

You would be right if you chose chi-square. And as a reward you are going to get your first opportunity to try out a statistical test, namely the aforementioned chi-square.

Trying out your first inferential statistical test: chi-square

By now we can tell that you are itching to try out your first statistical test. All this speculation regarding using statistical tests isn't as exciting as doing it for real. So let us try one. In this section we introduce you to your first statistical test: the chi-square.

● The chi-square test

As you know from the last exercise, the **chi-square** test provides a test for use when a researcher wants to examine the relationship between two categorical-type variables. For example, if we had two variables, Sex of Respondent and Type of Work Performed by the Respondent (full- and part-time work), we would be able to examine whether the two variables are associated. Often, people think that men tend to have full-time jobs and women tend to have part-time jobs. This type of thinking might be a research question. That is, is there a relationship between the variables? Does the sex of the respondent tend to determine what sort of work they undertake?

The key idea underlying the chi-square test is that we examine two sets of frequencies: observed and expected. To illustrate this, let us take the everyday example of men and women in full- and part-time work. Table 6.2 sets out these two aspects: observed and, in brackets, expected frequencies. The researcher, interested in whether the sex of a person influences the type of work they engage in, has asked 100 respondents their sex and whether they were employed in full-time or part-time work. The chi-square test analyses a matrix (often referred to as cross-tabulations) made up of cells representing each of the possible combinations of the levels of each categorical-type variable, in this case males and full-time work, females and full-time work, males and part-time work, and females and part-time work. As you can see from the table, there are two possible sets of frequencies.

The first set of numbers is the **observed frequencies**. These are an example of a set of frequencies the researcher might have found having gone out and collected the data from 100 people (Males and full-time work = 40, Females and full-time work = 10, Males and part-time work = 10, and Females and part-time work = 40).

The second set of numbers (in brackets) is the **expected frequencies**. These are the frequencies the researcher would expect to emerge from 100 people if everything was equal and, therefore, there was no association between the two variables. These frequencies are spread evenly across the possible combination of levels for each of the categorical-type variables (Males and full-time work = 25, Females and part-time work = 25, Males and part-time work = 25, and Females and part-time work = 25).

The chi-square test uses significance testing to examine whether two variables are independent (sometimes the chi-square test is referred to as the test of independence). What this means is that if the two variables are independent of each other, that is, are not related, then the *observed* frequencies would be split pretty evenly across the different rows and columns of the cross-tabulation (much like the expected frequencies are). Using our example, if the two variables are independent of each other, that is, if sex has no bearing on the type of work a person does, then you would expect to find that the observed frequencies are evenly split across the matrix.

Table 6.2 Breakdown of 100 respondents by sex and type of work

	Full-time work	Part-time work
Males	40 (25)	10 (25)
Females	10 (25)	40 (25)

However, if the observed frequencies are not even across the matrix, and if certain levels of one variable went together with other aspects of the other variable more so than would be expected, then we might begin to think that the two variables are linked in some way.

This is what appears to be happening with the observed frequencies in our example of sex of respondent and type of work. In terms of frequencies, 40 males are in full-time work (whereas only 10 males are in part-time work), and 40 females are in part-time work (whereas only 10 females are in full-time work). Therefore, what we can see in these data is a tendency for men to be employed in full-time work and women to be employed in part-time work. This suggests that the two variables might not be independent of each other and may be related. This possible relationship within a chi-square is often referred to as an association (which is why you will also sometimes find the chi-square referred to as a test of association as well as a test of independence; don't worry though – just remember, if the variables are related then they are 'associated'; if they are not related they are 'independent'). The chi-square statistic allows us to determine whether there is a statistically significant association (relationship) between two variables.

A research example to which this type of test could be applied is that by Powell *et al.* (2004). Their study looked at different staff perceptions of community learning disability nurses' roles. One of the things that the researchers were interested in was whether health staff or social care staff were more likely to see assessment as part of the community learning disability nurses' role. Therefore, the study has two categorical-type variables:

- whether the respondent is health staff or social care staff;
- whether the respondent believes that it is the community learning disability nurses' role to carry out assessment.

A chi-square analysis here could help us find out whether there is an association between the type of staff (health or social) and their view on whether it is the community learning disability nurses' role to carry out assessment (or whether these two variables were independent of each other, that is, whether the type of staff had no bearing on their views of the learning disability nurses' role to carry out assessment).

Let us show you how to calculate the chi-square in SPSS for Windows.

● The chi-square test in SPSS for Windows

Let us illustrate how a chi-square works using the example we referred to in the previous exercise. Following efforts by NHS Lothian to combat the MRSA hospital superbug, your local health authority has decided to see whether the 40 hospitals under its administration could benefit from such a drive. Research staff at the local health authority have then surveyed each of the authority's hospitals on two issues:

- whether there have been any special initiatives within the hospital, such as information packs on infection control and prevention given to staff, or posters and leaflets aimed at patients and visitors to raise awareness of the problem? Responses are either yes or no;

- whether the hospital has been given a clean bill of health in terms of there not being a reported case of the MRSA hospital superbug in the hospital. Responses are either yes or no.

There is a special dataset (mrsa.sav) on the book's website at www.pearsoned.co.uk/maltby. Download this dataset and open it up. There are two variables in this dataset:

- **Initiative**, which refers to whether there have been any special initiatives in the hospital (0 = No, 1 = Yes).

- **FreeofMRSA**, which refers to whether the hospital has been given a clean bill of health in terms of there not being a reported case of the MRSA superbug in the hospital (0 = No, 1 = Yes).

Click on the **Analyze** pull-down menu, click on **Descriptive Statistics**, and then click on **Crosstabs**. You will get a Window like that in Figure 6.7. Within the **Variables** box in the Crosstabs window, click on **Initiative** and then on the arrow button to move the variable into the **Row(s)** box. Click on **FreeofMRSA** and then on the arrow button to move the variable into the **Column(s)** box. Then click on the **Statistics...** box.

Click the box next to **Chi-square**. Click on **Continue**, and then hit **OK**. You should now get an output window like that in Figure 6.8.

In this output we have all the information we need to ascertain whether there is a statistically significant association between the launching of any special initiatives in the hospital and the absence of the MRSA superbug in the hospital.

The next stage is to report these statistics. There is a formal way of doing this. An important rule to remember when interpreting and writing tests is to *describe* and then *decide*. In other words, describe what is happening within the findings, and then decide whether the result is statistically significant.

Using 'describe and decide' to interpret the chi-square test

From the output in Figure 6.8, you will need to consider the following:

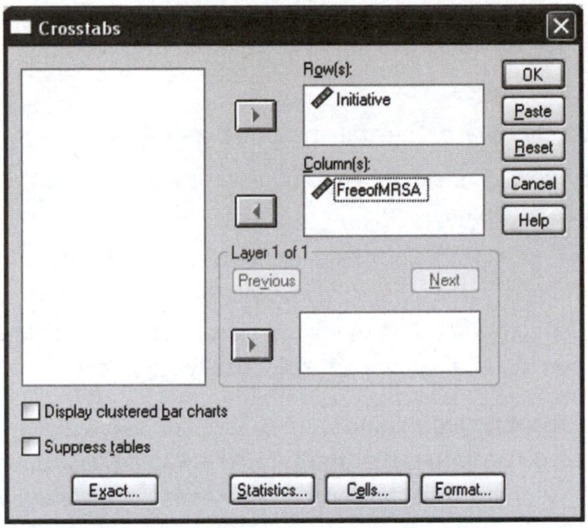

Figure 6.7 *Crosstabs window*

Initiative * FreeofMRSA Crosstabulation

		FreeofMRSA		Total
		No	Yes	
Initiative	No	15	6	21
	Yes	6	13	19
Total		21	19	40

← Frequency counts

Chi-Square Tests

	Value	df	Asymp. Sig. (2-sided)	Exact. Sig. (2-sided)	Exact. Sig. (1-sided)
Pearson Chi-Square	6.352(b)	1	.012		
Continuity Correction(a)	4.854	1	.028		
Likelihood Ratio	6.526	1	.011		
Fisher's Exact Test				.025	.013
Linear-by-Linear Association	6.193	1	.013		
N of Valid Cases	40				

a. Computed only for a 2 × 2 table
b. 0 cells (.0%) have expected count less than 5. The minimum expected count is 9.03.

Chi-square statistic   Significance level

Figure 6.8 *Chi-square output*

- *The breakdown of the values within the cells.* It is important here that you try to provide an overall picture of where most of the respondents, or not many of the respondents, are placed.
- *Pearson chi-square.* The statistical test statistic.
- *The Asymp. Sig. (2-sided).* The significance level. This is the probability level given to the current findings.
- *Whether the Asymp. Sig. (2-sided) figure suggests that the relationship between the two variables is statistically significant.* Remember, if this figure is below the $p = 0.05$ or $p = 0.01$ criterion then the finding is statistically significant. If this figure is above 0.05 then the findings are not statistically significant.

If we look at the upper box in Figure 6.8 we can see a general trend. The local authority sampled 40 hospitals; therefore if there was no association between the two variables, the hospitals would be divided fairly equally between each of the cells, giving ten in each. However, we can see a trend. The frequency counts are highest when:

- there were no special initiatives in the hospital; there has been a case of the MRSA in the hospital (15 cases).
- there has been a special initiative in the hospital; there has been no case of the MRSA in the hospital (13 cases).

However, the way to determine whether there is an association between hospital initiative and absence of the MRSA superbug is to use significance testing.

The significance level is $p = 0.012$. This is below the criterion of 0.05, and therefore we can conclude that there is a statistically significant relationship between hospital initiatives and whether the hospital is free of the MRSA superbug. In the present case, the trend we observe of frequency counts being weighted towards when there are no special initiatives in the hospital, there being a case of the MRSA in the hospital, and when there has been a special initiative in the hospital, there has been no case of the MRSA in the hospital, is found to be statistically significant. Therefore, there is an association between hospital initiatives to combat the MRSA superbug and the hospital being given a clean bill of health.

Using 'describe and decide' to report the chi-square test

The next stage is that you will need to report all the findings.

There is a formal way of reporting the chi-square. This comprises two elements. First, there is a formal statement of your statistics, which must include:

- *The test statistic.* Each test has a symbol for its statistic. The chi-square symbol is χ^2. Therefore, in your write-up you must include what χ^2 is equal to. In the example, $\chi^2 = 6.35$ (note that we reduce to two decimal places).

- *The degrees of freedom* (d.f.; to read more about these see Box 6.1). This is the number of rows minus 1, times the number of columns minus 1 (here [2 – 1] × [2 – 1] = 1 × 1 = 1). This is placed between the χ^2 and the equals sign and placed in brackets. Here, the degrees of freedom are 1. Therefore, $\chi^2(1) = 6.35$.

- *The probability*. This can be reported in two ways:

  - Traditionally this was done in relation to whether your probability value was below 0.05 or 0.01 (statistically significant) or above 0.05 (not statistically significant). Here, you use smaller than (<) or greater than (>) the criteria levels. You state these criteria by reporting whether $p < 0.05$ (statistically significant), $p < 0.01$ (statistically significant) or $p > 0.05$ (not statistically significant). So, in the example above, as $p = 0.012$, we would have written $p < 0.05$ and place this after the reporting of the χ^2 value. Therefore, $\chi^2(1) = 6.35$, $p < 0.05$.

  - More recently, statisticians and researchers have started reporting the p value as it is; in our case $p = 0.012$. We will use primarily this style throughout the book (though do not worry, we will keep reminding you of this distinction where appropriate). Therefore, in the present case we would write $\chi^2(1) = 6.35$, $p = 0.012$. It is important to note that practice varies, and your lecturers may insist on using the more traditional method, but today most disciplines suggest writing p as its actual value. What is important to note is that you still interpret the statistical significance of your findings in terms of its being greater or smaller than 0.05 and 0.01 – it's just that you report the actual probability value rather than use the < and > signs.

This must then be incorporated into a text, to help the reader understand and conceptualise your findings. In writing, the text uses the 'describe and decide' rule to inform your reader of your findings:

- Remind the reader of the two variables you are examining.
- Describe the relationship between the two variables in terms of the cell counts (and percentages).
- Tell the reader whether the finding is statistically significant or not.

You can use all the information above to write a fairly simple sentence, which conveys your findings succinctly but effectively. However, you will also need to include a table. Therefore, using the findings above we might report as follows:

Table 1 [see Figure 6.9] shows a breakdown of the distribution of respondents by each of the cells. The frequency of respondents in each cell was distributed such that the highest counts were for when there were no special initiatives in the hospital, there has been a case of the MRSA in the hospital (15 cases) and when there has been a special initiative in the hospital, there has been no case of the MRSA in the hospital (13 cases). A chi-square test was used to determine whether there was a statistically significant association between the two variables. A statistically

Box 6.1 Point to consider

What are degrees of freedom?

Whenever you use a statistical test you will always be asked to report your degrees of freedom. It is sometimes considered more a matter of convention than essential, but it is good practice to do it. This is always very straightforward and easy to do.

Many authors rightly shy away from explaining what degrees of freedom are. However, one of the best explanations of how to conceptualise degrees of freedom is presented by Clegg (1982). Here, Clegg suggests you imagine two pots, one of coffee and one of tea, but neither is labelled. Clegg asks the question, 'How many tastes do you require before you know what is in each pot?'

The answer is one, because once you have tasted one, you not only know what is in that pot, but also what is in the other. Similarly, if you had three pots, coffee, tea and orange juice, you would need two tastes before you could conclude what was in all three pots. What is important here is that you *do not* need to taste all of the pots before you are certain what is in each pot.

These ideas are used in the measuring of variables. In both examples, all the pots represent your sample, and your tasting represents your sampling. Each pot-tasting represents another procedure to establish certainty for your findings. Further, your number of attempts will be one less than the total number of pots. Degrees of freedom can be visualised in the same way.

You will note with the inferential statistical tests that we introduce you to in this book that the degrees of freedom for any variable are the size of the sample minus either 1 or 2. We will tell you whether it is 1 or 2 as we encounter each test.

If you end up using the hand-worked examples in this book (see Box 6.5) then you will see why degrees of freedom are important: you use them to help you decide whether your result is statistically significant. However, you will not see this if you are using SPSS for Windows as the program does all the calculations automatically.

significant association was found between the presence of initiatives and the hospital being given a clean bill of health with regard to the MRSA superbug ($\chi^2(1) = 6.35$, $p = 0.012$). The present findings suggest that initiatives to combat the MRSA superbug in hospitals are related to the hospital's reporting no cases of MRSA in their hospital.

Table 1: Breakdom of sample by initiatives in place in hospitals and reporting of the MRSA superbug

		FreeofMRSA		
		No	Yes	Total
Initiative	No	15	6	21
	Yes	6	13	19
Total		21	19	40

Figure 6.9 *Example of table for reporting the chi-square test*

Box 6.2 Point to consider

Relationships do not represent causation

It is important to remember, when reporting any sort of relationship, not to infer that one variable *causes* another. Sometimes it may be obvious that one variable causes another; for example, in the sex differences in choice of type of work, it is obvious that sex is influential in the type of work that people end up in, because there is no way that your choice of work can influence what sex you are. However, more often you need to think about it more carefully, and to choose your words cautiously when discussing relationships. With the MRSA example above, we could *not* conclude that special initiatives in the hospital causes there to be no cases of the MRSA superbug, as it may be that those hospitals that are found to be cleaner (and hence have no MRSA) are also hospitals that are more likely to run initiatives that encourage even greater levels of hygiene. Therefore it is more likely that the two variables influence each other and/or work together. Therefore, always remember when you are discussing your two variables to talk about 'relationships' between them, and not to say that one variable causes the other, unless you have a very good reason for thinking so.

You will of course find different ways of writing up the chi-square statistic, both in your own reports and in those of other authors, but you will find all the information included above in each write-up. Read Boxes 6.2-6.4 for further points to consider when using chi-square.

Box 6.3 Point to consider

Writing up a statistically non-significant result for the chi-square test: an example

The table below shows a breakdown of the distribution of respondents by each of the cells. The frequency of respondents in each cell was distributed evenly across the categories. A chi-square test was used to determine whether there was a statistically significant association between the two variables. No statistically significant association was found between presence of initiatives and the hospital being given a clean bill of health with regard to the MRSA superbug ($\chi^2(1) = 1.05$, $p = 0.78$). The present findings suggest that there is no association between initiatives to combat the MRSA superbug in hospitals and a hospital's reporting cases of MRSA in it, and that the two variables are independent of each other.

		Free of MRSA?		
		No	Yes	Total
Initiative	No	9	9	18
	Yes	11	11	22
Total		20	20	40

Box 6.4 Point to consider

Further information on the chi-square test

There are two conditions under which it is not advisable to do a chi-square test:

● When you have a chi-square that comprises two rows by two columns and any of the expected frequencies is less than 5.

● When you have a chi-square that comprises more than two rows by two columns and any of the expected frequencies is less than 1, or more than 20 per cent of the expected frequencies are less than 5.

Box 6.5 Point to consider

Calculating the chi-square by hand

Throughout this book we are going to give you the chance to see how these statistical tests work by the actual calculations. Although it is perfectly adequate just to perform these tests in SPSS for Windows, some people gain a clearer understanding of the statistic by working through the hand calculation. So there is a series of Point to consider boxes that allow you to work through the tests by hand. This one is for calculating the chi-square statistic.

New figures on heart disease indicate a stark divide between the number of sufferers in Glasgow and Edinburgh (http://news.bbc.co.uk/1/hi/scotland/ 4351554.stm). The Scottish Executive figures show that, despite improvement across the country, the three areas suffering most coronary heart disease are in Glasgow and that people in those areas are twice as likely to suffer from heart disease as in the more prosperous areas of Edinburgh. Researchers are interested in seeing whether they can replicate the findings. They have collected data among 100 respondents on two categorical variables: whether the person lives in Glasgow or Edinburgh, and whether they have been diagnosed with heart disease. Let us examine whether there is an association between area of residence and having heart disease.

	No heart disease	Heart disease	Row totals
Edinburgh	32 (A: Step 1)	15 (B: Step 1)	47 (Step 2)
Glasgow	20 (C: Step 1)	33 (D: Step 1)	53 (Step 2)
Column and row total	52 (Step 3)	48 (Step 3)	Overall total = 100 (Step 4)

Step 1. Name each of the cells:

$32 = A$, $15 = B$, $20 = C$, $33 = D$

Step 2. Work out the total for each of the rows:

$32 + 15 = 47$, $20 + 33 = 53$

Step 3. Work out the total for each of the columns:

$32 + 20 = 52$, $15 + 33 = 48$

Step 4. Work out the total for all the cells:

$32 + 15 + 20 + 33 = 100$

Step 5. Work out expected frequency for each of the cells, by multiplying its row total by its column total divided by the total for the sample:

A: $47 \times 52/100 = 24.44$

B: $47 \times 48/100 = 22.56$

C: $53 \times 52/100 = 27.56$

D: $53 \times 48/100 = 25.44$

	Observed	Expected (step 5)	Step 6	Step 7	Step 8
A	32	24.44	7.56	57.1536	2.339
B	15	22.56	−7.56	57.1536	2.533
C	20	27.56	−7.56	57.1536	2.074
D	33	25.44	7.56	57.1536	2.247

Step 6. Subtract expected frequency from the observed value:

A: $32 - 24.44 = 7.56$

B: $15 - 22.56 = -7.56$

C: $20 - 27.56 = -7.56$

D: $33 - 25.44 = 7.56$

Step 7. Square each of the values obtained in step 6. Each is 57.1536.

Step 8. Divide your finding for step 7 by your finding for each cell in step 5 (to three decimal places).

A: $57.1536/24.44 = 2.339$

B: $57.1536/22.56 = 2.533$

C: $57.1536/27.56 = 2.074$

D: $57.1536/25.44 = 2.247$

Step 9. Add up all the scores for all your cells in step 8.

$2.339 + 2.533 + 2.074 + 2.247 = 9.193$. This is your chi-square statistic.

Step 10. Work out your degrees of freedom by multiplying (number of rows −1) by (number of colums −1) = $(2 - 1) \times (2 - 1) = 1 \times 1 = 1$.

Step 11. Look at row in the table below and find the value that the chi-square is bigger than. Here it is bigger than 6.64, so our finding is significant at the 0.001 level.

	Significance levels for one-tailed test			
	0.05	0.025	0.01	0.005
	Significance levels for two-tailed test			
d.f.	0.10	0.05	0.02	0.01
1	2.71	3.84	5.41	6.64
2	4.60	5.99	7.82	9.21
3	6.25	7.82	9.84	11.34
4	7.78	9.49	11.67	13.28

Summary

You have been introduced to probability, significance, inferential statistics, decision making and your first statistical test, the chi-square. If it has all been a little overwhelming, do not worry – we will be revisiting many of these points again and again in the next two chapters as we introduce you to all the tests.

You are now able to:

✔ outline what is meant by terms such as distribution, probability and statistical significance testing;

✔ outline the importance of probability values in determining statistical significance;

✔ outline the decision-making process about what informs the use of parametric and non-parametric statistical tests;

✔ determine a statistically significant result;

✔ carry out the chi-square statistical test.

In the next chapter we are going to introduce you to two more statistical tests which form what is known as correlation statistics.

Self-assessment exercise

In the following exercises we are going to test your knowledge of descriptive statistics by exploring the nursing branch datasets. Select a dataset that is appropriate to your branch of nursing and load it up. For your dataset, answer the corresponding questions. Guidance for, and answers to, these questions are provided on the book's website at www.pearsoned.co.uk/maltby.

Adult branch

In 2003, Colin Perdue published an article suggesting that falls not only were a consequence of aging but also might be caused by a number of risk factors coming together, one of these being environmental factors such as tripping over something at home, or bumping into something, or losing one's balance (Perdue, 2003). Let us consider this idea of factors coming together with two variables in the adult branch dataset: (1) whether the fall was the result of an environmental factor (**environmentalfall**) and (2) whether the person has visual impairment (**visimpair**). Using this dataset, find out whether there is a statistically significant association between the patient being visually impaired and whether the fall was the result of an environmental factor.

Mental health branch

This exercise reflects the findings of Frances Forde *et al.* (2005) who examined the relationship between the number of psychological treatment sessions completed by patients (one to five sessions, six to eight sessions) and the change in self-rated depressive and anxiety symptoms. Forde *et al.* found that individuals who fell into the six to eight psychological treatment sessions were at an optimal level for their treatment, which suggests that it is at this level that treatment has been most effective.

In our data we have sought to examine this finding. We have measured the number of psychological treatment sessions each person has had and have created a variable that splits the sample into those who have had between one and five sessions and those who have had between six and eight sessions (**categorysession**). Our second variable reflects an assessment of the patient's doctor as to whether the person requires more psychological treatment sessions (**needfurthersessions**). Using this dataset, find out whether there is a statistically significant association between the category that the person falls into for the number of treatment sessions and the assessment of the patient's doctor as to whether the person requires more psychological treatment sessions.

Learning disability branch

This exercise reflects the findings made by Lisa Goodman and E. Keeton (2005) who discussed how choice of diet with learning disability may underlie a number of problems with learning, including encouraging passivity and discouraging independence. Causes of lack of choice in diet might result from environmental factors (group living, service structures and resource limitations), staff behaviour or the individual's own difficulties (such as having limited experience of making choices).

In this sample we are going to look at this basic idea and at the relationship made between two assessments by the nurse: whether the individual makes active choices over their food (**activechoice**) and whether they show independence (**independence**). Looking at these variables, determine whether there is a statistically significant association between individuals making active choices over their food and whether they show independence.

Child branch

Linda Diggle (2005) published an article about understanding and dealing with parental vaccine concerns. In this article she highlights the issues that commonly concern parents and suggests appropriate information that nurses can give to reassure parents and to promote vaccination.

In this dataset we want to find out whether there is an association between whether our mothers are first-time mothers (**firstch**) and whether they voiced concerns to our nurse over vaccines (**vaccineconcern**). Looking at these variables, determine whether there is a statistically significant association between whether the mother is a first-time mother and whether the mothers have concerns over vaccines.

Further reading

We would encourage you to read the articles mentioned in the self-assessment section to develop ideas around these topics. They are all available free online (after registering) at the *Nursing Times* website: www.nursingtimes.net/.
The references for the articles are:

Diggle, L. (2005) 'Understanding and dealing with parental vaccine concerns', *Nursing Times* 101(46): 26–28.

Forde, F. *et al.* (2005) 'Optimum number of sessions for depression and anxiety', *Nursing Times*, 101(43): 36–40.

Goodman, L. and Keeton, E. (2005) 'Choice in the diet of people with learning difficulties', *Nursing Times* 101(14): 28–29.

Perdue, C. (2003) 'Falls in older people: taking a multidisciplinary approach', *Nursing Times* 99(31): 28–30.

You will be able to access the articles by typing the first author's surname or the title of the paper in the Search box on the website.

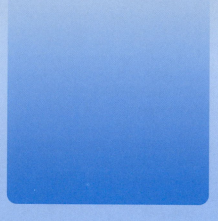

Chapter 7

Correlational statistics

Key themes

✔ Correlations

✔ Pearson product-moment correlation coefficient

✔ Spearman's rho correlation coefficient

Learning outcomes

By the end of this chapter you will have learnt the rationale for, the procedure for and the interpretation in SPSS for Windows of two inferential statistical tests:

✔ Pearson product-moment correlation

✔ Spearman's rho correlation

Introduction

Imagine . . . That you are a nurse working in a younger disabled unit (YDU) with patients who have physical disabilities. You want to examine whether there is a relationship between how often the patients in the YDU carry out exercise and the level of bodily pain that they experience. You decide to carry out a project into pain and exercise among these patients and you ask them to complete a questionnaire designed to assess their quality of life: the SF-36 Health Survey. This questionnaire enables you to measure frequency of exercise and bodily pain among the patients as it naturally occurs. You are not introducing anything to change the patients' levels of bodily pain or their exercise. You are merely seeing whether there is a relationship between these two variables and, if so, how strong the relationship is. Such information will help to inform any attempts that you might want to make to increase a patient's level of physical exercise, but first you need to see whether the two variables are related. We shall be revisiting the use of this quality-of-life questionnaire later in this chapter.

In Chapter 6 we introduced you to your first inferential statistical test: the chi-square. What we intend to do now is to build on your knowledge by introducing you to two more tests. Cast your mind back to the decision-making table presented in Figure 6.6. Now look at Figure 7.1. When using this there was a section that related to having two separate continuous variables to examine. The Pearson and Spearman statistics are two statistics that you use when you want to examine the relationship between two separate continuous-type variables. The Pearson correlation statistical test is a parametric statistical test (you remember when your data show a normal distribution and are not skewed). The Spearman correlation statistical test is a non-parametric statistical test (when your data are not normally distributed or you find evidence of their being skewed). We will next introduce you to the thinking that lies behind these two statistical tests.

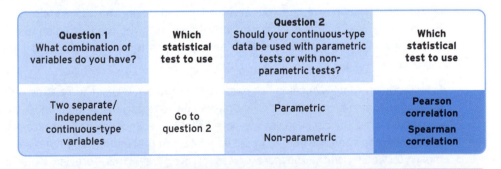

Question 1 What combination of variables do you have?	Which statistical test to use	Question 2 Should your continuous-type data be used with parametric tests or with non-parametric tests?	Which statistical test to use
Two separate/ independent continuous-type variables	Go to question 2	Parametric Non-parametric	Pearson correlation Spearman correlation

Figure 7.1 The part of the decision-making table (Figure 6.6) that relates to correlation statistics

Energiser

Before you start we are going to get your brain warmed up mathematically and get you to carry out some simple calculations (see Figure 7.2). Although these calculations may seem rather simple and redundant, they are related to some of the concepts you will come across in the chapter and will help your understanding.

What is a correlation?

The aim of both the Pearson and Spearman correlation coefficients is to determine whether there is a relationship between two separate continuous-type variables.

Imagine two variables: *amount of chocolate eaten* and *weight*. It is thought that chocolate contains a lot of fat, and that eating a lot of fat will increase your weight. Therefore, it could be expected that people who eat a lot of chocolate would also weigh a lot. If this were true then the amount of chocolate you eat and your weight would be *positively correlated*. The more chocolate you eat, the more you weigh. The less chocolate you eat, the less you weigh. This is a correlation, but this is a positive correlation, because when the scores are high on one continuous-type variable, they are high on the other continuous-type variable (and low scores on one are accompanied by low scores on the other). This is visualised in Figure 7.3(a), with the plotted points moving from the lower left-hand corner up and across to the upper right-hand corner of the chart.

Conversely, a negative correlation between two variables is the opposite of that: a high negative correlation would mean that while scores on one variable rise, scores on the other variable decrease. An example of this would be the amount of exercise taken and weight. It is thought that taking exercise will usually lead to a decrease in weight. If this were true then the amount of exercise you take and your weight would be negatively correlated. The more exercise you take, the less you weigh. The less exercise you take, the more you weigh. This is visualised in Figure 7.3(b), with the plotted points moving from the upper left-hand corner down and across to the lower right-hand corner of the chart.

Finally, some variables might not be expected to show any level of correlation with each other. For example, the number of hot meals you have eaten and the number of times you have visited the zoo. Usually, we expect that there would be no logical reason why eating hot meals and zoo visiting would be related, so that eating more hot meals would mean you would visit the zoo more, or less (or vice versa). Therefore, you would expect the number of hot meals you have eaten and the number of times you have visited the zoo *not* to show any correlation. This is visualised in Figure 7.3(c) by a random scatter of plots; the plots show no clear direction, going neither up nor down.

Energiser 1

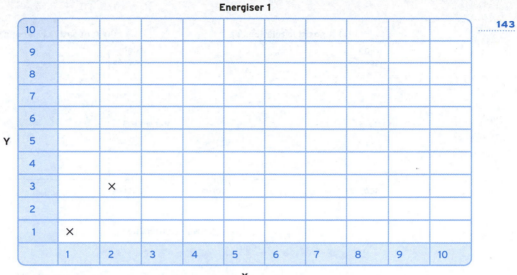

Plot each combination of numbers (X, Y) on the grid above. We have done the first two for you.

X	1	2	3	4	5	6	8	8	9	10
Y	1	3	2	4	6	7	8	9	9	10

Energiser 2

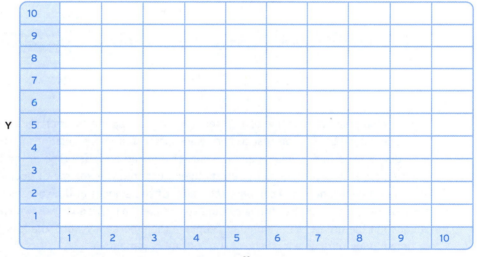

Now plot each combination of numbers (X, Y) on the grid above.

X	10	9	8	4	5	6	3	3	2	1
Y	1	2	2	4	5	4	7	8	9	10

Figure 7.2 *Energiser*

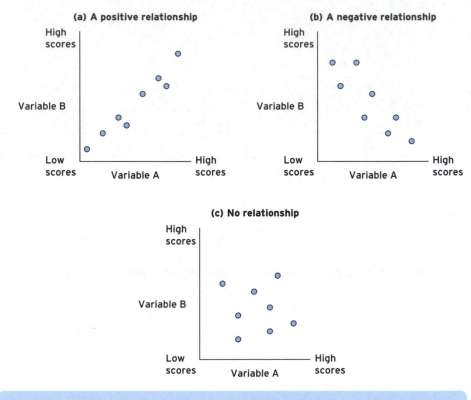

Figure 7.3 *Examples of positive, negative and no relationships between two variables*

One nursing research example of a correlation was carried out by Cherri Hobgood and her colleagues (2005). The researchers were interested in the relationship between emergency department volume and the impact this had on nurse time at the bedside in an emergency department. Therefore, they measured the volume of people in the emergency department and compared this against the amount of time nurses spent at the patients' bedsides. They found a negative correlation between these two variables, suggesting the greater the volume of people in the emergency ward, the less amount of time nurses were able to spend at the bedside of patients.

● Scatterplot

You can represent correlational relationships through the use of scatterplots on SPSS for Windows. Scatterplots are graphs that plot scores for one variable against the scores on another variable, like those in Figure 7.3. Let us quickly try one. Load up SPSS for Windows, and load up the child branch dataset. Now, in this dataset there are two

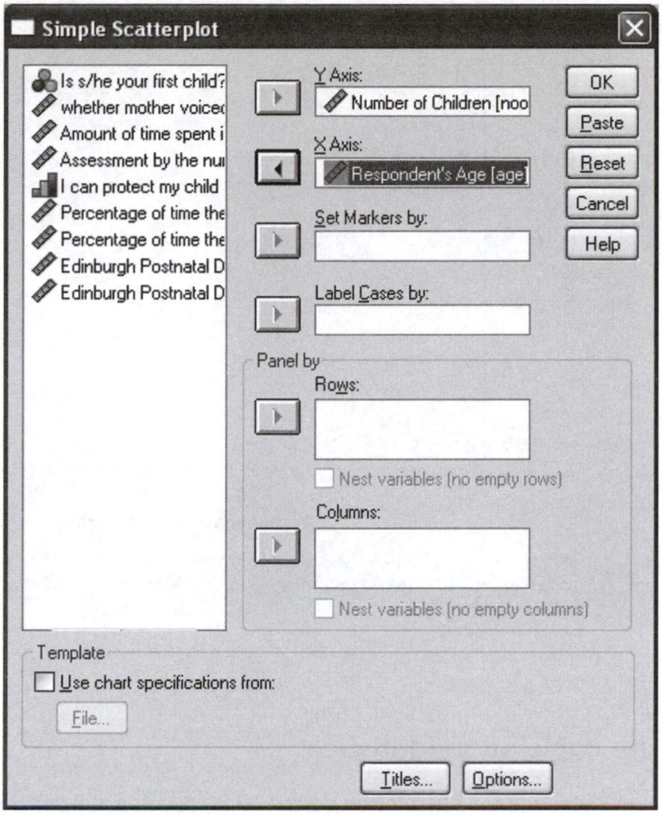

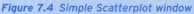

Figure 7.4 *Simple Scatterplot window*

variables: age of the respondent (**age**) and number of children that the respondent has (**noofChild**). Now, you would perhaps expect that these two variables, if put into a scattergram, would show a positive correlation between the variables, because the older you are the more likely you are to have had more children.

To do a scatterplot in SPSS for Windows, click on **Graphs** and then click on **Scatter/ dot…** . The box surrounding **Simple Scatter** should be highlighted. Now click on **Define**. Transfer the number of children variable (**NoofChild**) variable into the **Y axis** box, and the age variable (**age**) into the **X axis** box (see Figure 7.4). Then press **OK**. You should get a figure like that in Figure 7.5.

You will see that, generally, the scatterplot is in a positive direction, with low values on one variable being accompanied by low values on the other variable, and high values on one variable accompanied by high values on the other.

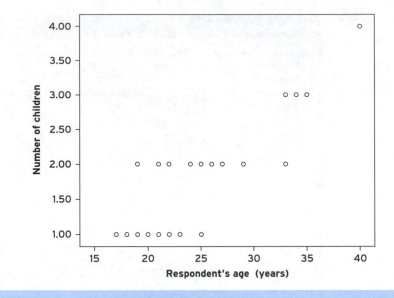

Figure 7.5 *Scatterplot between respondents' ages and the number of children they have*

The correlation statistic

We now know what a correlation generally is, and the description of the relationship, but so far we have vague information. However, the Pearson and Spearman correlation statistics can give us much more information. The correlation coefficient provides a statistic that tells us the direction, the strength and the significance of the relationship between two variables.

What do we mean by direction and strength? Well, both the **Pearson** and **Spearman correlation statistics** use the number of the data and present a final figure that indic-ates the direction and strength of the relationship. This final figure is always known as the correlation coefficient and is represented by *r* (Pearson) or *rho* (Spearman). The correlation coefficient will always be a value ranging from +1.00 through 0.00 to –1.00.

- A correlation of +1.00 would be a 'perfect' positive relationship.
- A correlation of –1.00 would be a 'perfect' negative relationship.
- A correlation of 0.00 would be no relationship (no single straight line can sum up the almost random distribution of points).

All correlations, then, will range from –1.00 to +1.00. So a correlation statistic could be –0.43 (a negative relationship) or 0.53 (a positive relationship). It could be 0.01, close to no relationship. This figure can then be used with significance testing, such as the chi-square, to see whether the relationship between the two variables is statistically significant. Let us show you how one of these correlational statistics works.

Pearson product–moment correlation

Remember from Figure 7.1 that the Pearson product-moment correlation is a test used with parametric data, and is used when you have two continuous-type variables that you believe should be used in a parametric test (for example, it shows a normal distribution, or rather that the date are not skewed). Remember, too, that the key idea of the correlation statistical test is to determine whether there is a relationship between the two variables.

● Performing the Pearson product–moment correlation on SPSS for Windows

In the following example we will show how a Pearson product-moment correlation works by using some of the data from the adult branch dataset. One aspect of these data looks at the relationship between four dimensions of physical health as measured by the SF-36 Health Survey, Version 2 (Ware *et al.*, 1994, 2000). This questionnaire is a well-known and well-used multi-purpose short-form measure of general health status. The SF-36 includes four multi-item scales measuring:

- physical functioning – higher scores on this variable indicate worsened physical functioning (**physfunc**);
- role limitations due to physical health problems – higher scores on this variable indicate greater limitations to roles due to physical health problems (**Rolephys**);
- bodily pain – higher scores on this variable indicate a greater amount of bodily pain (**BodPain**);
- general heath perceptions – higher scores on this variable indicate a poorer perception of one's own general health (**genHealth**).

For this example we are going to use two of these four subscales to demonstrate a Pearson product-moment correlation coefficient. These are physical functioning (**physfunc**) and perception of one's own general health (**genHealth**). Generally, we would expect a statistically significant positive correlation between these two variables, given that poorer physical functioning might be the result of, or influence, feelings of general health. You might be feeling less healthy because you are poor in your physical functioning. You might feel less able to physically function because you are poor in your general health. Using the current dataset we will examine whether a statistically significant positive correlation occurs between these two variables.

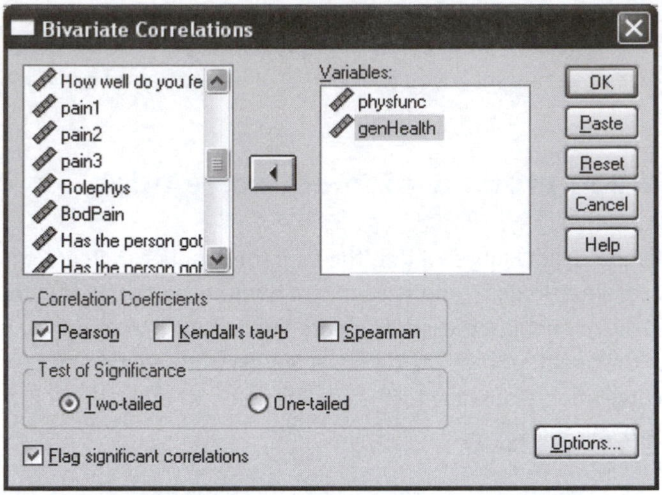

Figure 7.6 *Bivariate Correlations window*

Load up the adult dataset. Pull down the **Analyze** menu, choose **Correlate** and then **Bivariate**. The window shown in Figure 7.6 will come up. Then select the two variables we wish to correlate (**physfunc** and **genHealth**) by transferring their names into the **Variables:** box using the arrow button on the screen.

Click **Pearson** in the **Correlation Coefficients** box, and click the **Two-tailed** radio button in the **Test of Significance** box (see why in Box 7.1). Then run the correlation by clicking on **OK**. You will get an output which looks like Figure 7.7.

This output (Figure 7.7) contains all the information we need for an interpretation of whether there is a relationship between physical functioning and general health. The

Correlations

		physfunc	genHealth	
physfunc	Pearson Correlation	1	.356**	Correlation coefficient
	Sig. (2-tailed)		.002	
	N	74	74	Significance level
genHealth	Pearson Correlation	.356**	1	
	Sig. (2-tailed)	.002		
	N	74	74	

** Correlation is significant at the 0.01 level (2-tailed).

Figure 7.7 *Pearson product-moment correlation output between physical functioning and general health*

Box 7.1 Point to consider

One- and two-tailed hypotheses and significance testing

One-tailed and two-tailed tests involve making statements regarding the expected direction of the relationship between the two variables you are measuring. With a one-tailed **hypothesis** the researcher would make a statement regarding the specific direction of the relationship. With a two-tailed statement, prediction is not made regarding the direction of the expected relationship. We can illustrate this with the present example because we believe there is going to be a statistically significant *positive* (this is the expected direction of the relationship) relationship between physical functioning and bodily pain. A two-tailed hypothesis may be that we might expect a significant relationship, but we are unsure of the final direction of the relationship (here, the researcher would state that there is an expected statistically significant relationship between the two variables). As we can see from the present example, by making a specific prediction about the direction of the relationship between these aspects of physical health these ideas are incorporated into statistical significance testing, and we would use a one-tailed test.

In reality you are more likely to get a statistically significant result using a one-tailed test because the way the significance testing is set up allows you more leeway because you have made a prediction. This increases your chances of a statistically significant finding; it also increases your chances of making an error by suggesting there is a statistically significant relationship between two variables when in fact there is no such relationship (this is known as a Type I error). In nursing, it is crucial to avoid making this sort of mistake. You don't want to say a drug has a statistically significant effect when it doesn't. Therefore, many researchers don't make this distinction any more and tend to use two-tailed tests regardless of *a priori* predictions. Therefore, in future you might be best advised always to perform the correlations using the two-tailed test.

important rule to remember when interpreting and writing test results is to *describe* and then *decide*. In other words, describe what is happening within the findings, and then decide whether the result is statistically significant.

Using 'describe and decide' to interpret the Pearson product–moment correlation

From the output, you will need to consider three things:

- *Pearson correlation.* The statistical test statistic. It is important to note whether the statistic is positive or negative. This indicates whether the relationship between the two variables is positive (positive number, though SPSS doesn't print a + sign) or negative (represented by a − sign).

- *The Sig. (2-tailed).* The significance level. This is the probability level given to the current findings.

- *Whether the Sig. (2-tailed) figure suggests that the relationship between the two variables is statistically significant.* Remember, if this figure is below the $p = 0.05$ or $p = 0.01$ criterion, then the finding is statistically significant. If this figure is above 0.05, then the findings are not statistically significant.

The correlation between physical functioning (**physfunc**) and perception of general health (**genHealth**) is 0.356. This tells us that there is a positive relationship between the two variables. The poorer the physical functioning, the poorer the feeling of general health, and vice versa. If the relationship was a negative one, the statistic would have a minus sign in front of it. The significance level is $p = 0.002$, which is below the level of $p = 0.05$ or $p = 0.01$, so we can decide that the relationship we have found is not likely to have occurred by chance. Therefore, we can conclude that there is a statistically significant positive relationship between physical functioning and general heath.

Using 'decide and describe' to report the Pearson product–moment correlation

The next stage is to report these statistics. There is a formal way of reporting the Pearson product-moment correlation coefficient, which comprises two elements. The first element is that a formal statement of your statistics must include the following:

- *The test statistic.* Each test has a symbol for its statistic. The Pearson product-moment correlation has the symbol r. Therefore, in writing your results you must include what r is equal to. In the example, $r = 0.356$.

- *The degrees of freedom.* This is a figure that is traditionally reported (though it is worth noting that it is not always reported). For the Pearson product-moment correlation coefficient, the degrees of freedom equal the size of your sample minus 2. The minus 2 represents minus 1 for each set of scores (the set of scores for physical functioning scale and the set of scores for the general health scale). The figure is placed between the r and the equals sign and is written in brackets. Here, the degrees of freedom are 72 (size of sample = 74, minus 2 = 72). Therefore, $r(72) = 0.356$.

- *The probability.* You may remember from Chapter 6 that this is reported in one of two ways:

  - Traditionally, this was done in relation to whether your probability value was below 0.05 or 0.01 (statistically significant) or above 0.05 (not statistically significant). Here, you use less than (<) or greater than (>) the criteria levels.

You state these criteria by reporting whether $p < 0.05$ (statistically significant), $p < 0.01$ (statistically significant) or $p > 0.05$ (not statistically significant). In the example above, as $p = 0.004$ we would write $p < 0.01$ and place this after the reporting of the r value. Therefore, with our findings, $r(72) = 0.356$, $p < 0.01$.

- More recently, statisticians and researchers have started reporting the p value as it is; in our case $p = 0.004$. We will use primarily this style throughout the book (though do not worry we will keep reminding you of this distinction where appropriate). Therefore, in the present case we would write $r(72) = 0.356$, $p = 0.004$. It is important to note that practice varies, and your lecturers may insist on using the more traditional method, but today most disciplines suggest writing p as its actual value. What is important to note is that you still interpret the statistical significance of your findings in terms of it being greater or smaller than 0.05 and 0.01, it's just that you report the actual probability value rather than use the $<$ and $>$ signs.

The second element is the incorporation of these statistics into the text, to help the reader understand and interpret your findings. In writing the text, use the 'describe and decide' rule to inform the reader of your findings:

- Remind the reader of the two variables you are examining.
- Describe the relationship between the two variables as positive or negative.
- Tell the reader whether the finding is statistically significant or not.
- Give some indication of what this means.

Box 7.2 Point to consider

Writing up a statistically non-significant result for the Pearson product-moment correlation

Knowing how to write a statistically significant result is of little use if, in your research, you have a statistically non-significant finding. Therefore, whenever we suggest how you might report test results, we will also give you the alternative way of writing up your results. Here, let us imagine that we found no statistically significant relationship between physical functioning and bodily pain, i.e. $r = 0.032$ and $p = 0.76$ (therefore $p > 0.05$ and is statistically non-significant).

A Pearson product moment correlation coefficient was used to examine the relationship between physical functioning and general health using the subscales from the SF-36 Health Survey. No statistically significant correlation was found between physical functioning and general heath ($r(72) = 0.032$, $p = 0.76$), suggesting no statistically significant relationship between physical functioning and general health.

You can use all the information above to write a fairly simple sentence which conveys your findings succinctly but effectively. Therefore, using the findings above, we might report:

> A Pearson product-moment correlation coefficient was used to examine the relationship between physical functioning and general health using the subscales from the SF-36 Health Survey. A statistically significant positive correlation was found between physical functioning and general health ($r(72) = 0.356$, $p = 0.004$), suggesting that poorer physical functioning and general health are statistically significantly related to one another.

You will come across different ways of writing up the Pearson product-moment correlation coefficient, both in your own writing and in that of other authors, but you will find all the information included above in any write-up. Read Boxes 7.2 and 7.3 for further point to consider when using a Pearson product-moment correlation.

Box 7.3 Point to consider

Computing the Pearson product-moment correlation by hand

The following example reflects a study that tried to examine the relationship between physical functioning and general health. The study used established scales among a non-clinical sample of five respondents. The aim of the study was to see whether poorer levels of physical functioning are accompanied by poor levels of general health.

Respondent	Physical functioning score	General health score	Physical functioning squared	General health squared	Physical functioning by general health
1	5	4	25 (Step 1)	16 (Step 2)	20 (Step 3)
2	1	2	1 (Step 1)	4 (Step 2)	2 (Step 3)
3	1	1	1 (Step 1)	1 (Step 2)	1 (Step 3)
4	5	5	25 (Step 1)	25 (Step 2)	25 (Step 3)
5	3	3	9 (Step 1)	9 (Step 2)	9 (Step 3)

Step 1. Square each of the scores for the physical functioning variable:

$5 \times 5 = 25$, $1 \times 1 = 1$, $1 \times 1 = 1$, $5 \times 5 = 25$, $3 \times 3 = 9$

Step 2. Square each of the scores for the general health variable:

$4 \times 4 = 16$, $2 \times 2 = 4$, $1 \times 1 = 1$, $5 \times 5 = 25$, $3 \times 3 = 9$

Step 3. Multiply each of the scores for the physical functioning variable by each of the scores for the general health variable:

$5 \times 4 = 20$, $1 \times 2 = 2$, $1 \times 1 = 1$, $5 \times 5 = 25$, $3 \times 3 = 9$

Step 4. Add all the scores together for the physical functioning variable:

$5 + 1 + 1 + 5 + 3 = 15$

Step 5. Add all the scores together for the general health variable:

$4 + 2 + 1 + 5 + 3 = 15$

Step 6. Add all the scores together for the physical functioning variable squared (from step 1):

$25 + 1 + 1 + 25 + 9 = 61$

Step 7. Add all the scores together for the general health squared (from step 2):

$16 + 4 + 1 + 25 + 9 = 55$

Step 8. Add all the scores together for the physical functioning variable multiplied by general health variable from (step 3):

$20 + 2 + 1 + 25 + 9 = 57$

Step 9. Multiply your finding from step 8 by the number of people in the sample:

$57 \times 5 = 285$

Step 10. Multiply your finding from step 4 by your finding for step 5:

$15 \times 15 = 225$

Step 11. Subtract your finding from step 10 from your finding for step 9:

$285 - 225 = 60$

Step 12. Multiply your finding for step 6 by the number of people in the sample:

$61 \times 5 = 305$

Step 13. Square your finding for step 4:

$15 \times 15 = 225$

Step 14. Subtract your finding for step 13 from your finding for step 12:

$305 - 225 = 80$

Step 15. Multiply your finding for step 7 by the number of people in the sample:

$55 \times 5 = 275$

Step 16. Square your finding for step 5:

$15 \times 15 = 225$

Step 17. Subtract your finding for step 16 from your finding for step 15:

$275 - 225 = 50$

Step 18. Multiply your finding for step 14 by your finding for step 17:

$80 \times 50 = 4{,}000$

Step 19. Find the square root for step 18:

$\sqrt{4{,}000} = 63.245$

Step 20. Divide the finding for step 11 by the finding for step 19:

$60/63.245 = 0.949$

You should now have the value of $r = 0.949$.

You now have to determine whether the figure is statistically significant. Here, the procedure for all hand calculations is very different from using SPSS for Windows. You need to establish the significance level by comparing your test statistic with a predetermined number to see whether your result is statistically significant or not (this is not as exact as doing it on the computer because, remember, this was the system used before such calculations were possible on computer).

The first step is to determine the degrees of freedom (see Box 6.1 in Chapter 6 for an explanation of degrees of freedom). Degrees of freedom (d.f.) for the Pearson product–moment correlation coefficient are the size of sample minus 2 (with the minus 2 representing 1 for each set of scores). So in this case, $5 - 2 = 3$, d.f. = 3. You then determine the significance level for your test and choose either a one-tailed or two-tailed test and compare your r value with numbers on the table below.

We will use the $p = 0.05$ criterion and use a two-tailed statistic. The number that falls under d.f. = 3, $p = 0.05$ and use of two-tailed test is 0.8783. If your r figure is

• • •

higher (ignore whether the figure is + or –) than your d.f. figure then the relationship is statistically significant. On this occasion 0.949 (*r* figure) is higher than 0.8783 (d.f. figure). Therefore, Pearson's *r* is statistically significant here.

You now know your correlation statistic (*r*), whether your finding is statistically significant and, if it is, at what level it is statistically significant. You then write the Pearson product–moment correlation in the same way.

You must remember not to mix up the procedure for determining significance in hand calculation with the one for interpreting significance in SPSS for Windows, or else you will make mistakes in your reporting of statistics.

d.f. = *n* − 2	Significance levels for two-tailed test				
	0.10	0.05	0.02	0.01	0.001
	Significance levels for one-tailed test				
	0.05	0.025	0.01	0.005	0.0005
1	0.98769	0.99692	0.999507	0.999877	0.9999988
2	0.90000	0.95000	0.98000	0.990000	0.99900
3	0.8054	0.8783	0.93433	0.95873	0.99116
4	0.7293	0.8114	0.8822	0.91720	0.97406
5	0.6694	0.7545	0.8329	0.8745	0.95074

Spearman's rho correlation

The Spearman correlation is the non-parametric version of the parametric test the Pearson product–moment correlation. Whereas the Pearson product–moment correlation is used to examine whether a statistically significant relationship occurs between two continuous variables, which demonstrate properties suitable for use in parametric tests, the Spearman rho correlation is used to examine whether a statistically significant relationship occurs between two continuous variables, which demonstrate properties suitable for use in non-parametric tests. Apart from this, the Spearman rho correlation works in exactly the same way, but with a *rho* value between –1.00 and +1.00 being generated (though some people just use *r*). As with the Pearson correlation, significance testing is then used to determine whether a statistically significant relationship occurs between two variables.

● Performing the Spearman's rho correlation in SPSS for Windows

For this example we are going to use the other two variables from the SF-36 Health Survey:

● role limitations due to physical health problems – higher scores on this variable indicate greater limitations to roles due to physical health problems (**Rolephys**);

● bodily pain – higher scores on this variable indicate a greater amount of bodily pain (**BodPain**).

Before we confirm the use of these data in a non-parametric test, let us take a further look at these variables. Remember, one of the assumptions for parametric testing is that data demonstrate a normal distribution. So let us check we are right to put these two variables into a non-parametric test by looking at whether these data are skewed. Remember, data are skewed if the skewness statistic exceeds +1 or –1 (+1 being positively skewed and –1 being negatively skewed). Pull down the **Analyze** menu, select **Descriptive statistics** and click on **Descriptives**. Transfer variables **Rolephys** and **BodPain** into the **Variables** box. Then click on **Options** and click the **Skewness** box. Press **Continue** and then press **OK**. You should then get an output like that in Figure 7.8. (We have also produced the histograms to illustrate the skewness in the distribution of these variables, which you can perform if you prefer [detailed in Chapter 3] although this is not necessary as the skewness statistic gives you the information you need for deciding whether the data are skewed.)

From the table in Figure 7.8 you should see that both the skewness statistics are above the criterion 1 (be it positive or minus): **Rolephys** has a skewness of –1.519, and **BodPain** has a skewness of –1.038. This suggests that both these scales are skewed. Therefore, we might be wise to perform a non-parametric test with these data.

To compute and interpret the Spearman's rho correlation coefficient in SPSS for Windows, you generally do as you would for the calculation of the Pearson product–moment correlation coefficient. Pull down the **Analyze** menu, click on **Correlate**, then **Bivariate**. Transfer the two variables (**Rolephys** and **BodPain**) into the **Variables** box. However, in the **Correlation Coefficients** box (when choosing your variables), choose **Spearman** rather than **Pearson** in the bottom left-hand corner of the box. Press **OK** and you will get the output shown in Figure 7.9.

In this output we have all the information we need to interpret whether there is a relationship between role limitations due to physical health problems and bodily pain. The important rule to remember when interpreting and writing tests is to *describe* and then *decide*. In other words, describe what is happening within the findings, and then decide whether the result is statistically significant.

Descriptive Statistics

	N	Minimum	Maximum	Mean	Std.	Skewness	
	Statistic	Statistic	Statistic	Statistic	Statistic	Statistic	Std. Error
Rolephys	74	6.00	20.00	16.9189	3.53750	–1.519	.279
BodPain	74	2.00	11.00	8.3919	2.29244	–1.038	.279
Valid N (listwise)	74						

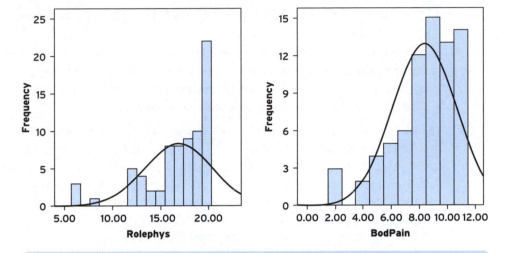

Figure 7.8 Descriptive statistics output (histograms, averages and dispersions) of role limitations due to physical health problems and bodily pain variables with skewness statistic

Correlations

			Rolephys	BodPain
Spearman's rho	Rolephys	Correlation Coefficient	1.000	.589**
		Sig. (2-tailed)	.	.000
		N	74	74
	BodPain	Correlation Coefficient	.589**	1.000
		Sig. (2-tailed)	.000	.
		N	74	74

Correlation coefficient

Significance level

**. Correlation is significant at the 0.01 level (2-tailed).

Figure 7.9 Spearman's rho output between role limitations due to physical health problems and bodily pain

Using 'describe and decide' to interpret the Spearman's rho correlation

From the output, you will need to consider three things;

- *Spearman's rho.* The statistical test. It is important to note whether the statistic is positive or minus. This indicates whether the relationship between the two variables is positive (positive number, though SPSS doesn't print a + sign) or negative (represented by a – sign).

- *The Sig. (2-tailed).* The significance level. This is the probability level given to the current findings.

- *Whether the Sig. (2-tailed) figure suggests that the relationship between the two variables is statistically significant.* Remember, if this figure is below the $p = 0.05$ or $p = 0.01$ criterion, then the finding is statistically significant. If this figure is above 0.05, then the findings are not statistically significant.

Therefore, the correlation between role limitations due to physical health problems (**Rolephys**) and bodily pain (**BodPain**) is $rho = 0.589$. This tells us that there is a positive relationship between role limitations due to physical health problems and bodily pain. The significance level is $p = 0.000$. This is below 0.01 so we can conclude that there is a statistically significant positive relationship between role limitations due to physical health problems and bodily pain. This means role limitations due to physical health problems in respondents are accompanied by bodily pain.

Using 'describe and decide' to report the Spearman's rho correlation

The next stage is to report these statistics. There is a formal way of reporting the Spearman's rho correlation which comprises two elements. First there is a formal statement of your statistics, and this must include the following:

- *The test statistic.* Each test has a symbol for its statistic. The Spearman's rho correlation uses the term *rho*. Therefore, in your write-up you must include what *rho* is equal to. In the example above $rho = 0.589$.

- *The degrees of freedom.* This concept was introduced in Chapter 6 and is usually reported when describing the results. For the Spearman's rho the degrees of freedom equal the size of your sample minus 2. Here, the minus 2 represents minus 1 for each set of scores (the set of scores for role limitations due to physical health problems and the set of scores for bodily pain). The figure is placed between the *rho* and the equals sign and is written in brackets. Here, the degrees of freedom are 72 (size of sample = 74, minus 2 = 72). Therefore, $rho(72) = 0.589$.

- *The probability.* You may remember from Chapter 6 that this is reported in one of two ways.

    - Traditionally, this was done in relation to whether your probability value was below 0.05 or 0.01 (statistically significant) or above 0.05 (not statistically significant).

Here, you use less than (<) or greater than (>) the criteria levels. You state these criteria by reporting whether $p < 0.05$ (statistically significant), $p < 0.01$ (statistically significant) or $p > 0.05$ (not statistically significant). In the example above, as $p = 0.000$ we would write $p < 0.01$ and place this after the reporting of the *rho* value. Therefore, with our findings, $rho(72) = 0.589$, $p < 0.01$.

- More recently, statisticians and researchers have started reporting the p value as it is; in our case $p = 0.000$. We will use primarily this style throughout the book (though do not worry – we will keep reminding you of this distinction where appropriate). Therefore, in the present case we would expect to write $rho(72) = 0.589$, $p = 0.000$. However, you need to bear in mind that the probability value that is reported as '.000' in SPSS appears as such because SPSS typically reports only to three decimal places, so actually '.000' means a value less than 0.0005. Consequently you would do better to report p as $p < 0.0005$. Finally, it is important to note that practice varies, and your lecturers may insist on using the more traditional method, but today most disciplines suggest writing p as its actual value. What is important to note is that you still interpret the statistical significance of your findings in terms of its being greater or less than 0.05 and 0.01; it's just that you report the actual probability value rather than use the < and > signs.

This must then be incorporated into the text to help the reader to understand and conceptualise your findings. In writing the text use the 'describe and decide rule' to inform the reader of your findings:

- Remind the reader of the two variables you are examining.
- Describe whether the relationship between the two variables is positive or negative.
- Tell the reader whether the finding is statistically significant or not.
- Give some indication of what this means.

You can use all the information above to write a fairly simple sentence which conveys your findings succinctly but effectively. Therefore, using the findings above we might report:

A Spearman's rho correlation was used to examine the relationship between role limitations due to physical health problems and bodily pain. A statistically significant positive correlation was found between role limitations due to physical health problems and bodily pain ($rho(72) = 0.589$, $p < 0.0005$), suggesting that role limitations and physical health problems accompany one another.

You will of course find different ways of writing up the Spearman's rho correlation both in your own writing and in that of other authors, but you will find all the information included above in any report. Read Boxes 7.4–7.6 for further points to consider when using a Spearman's rho correlation.

Box 7.4 Point to consider

Writing up a statistically non-significant result for the Spearman rho correlation

Let us imagine that we found no significant relationship between role limitations due to physical health problems and bodily pain, i.e. $rho = 0.030$, and $p = 0.56$ (therefore $p > 0.05$ and non-significant).

> A Spearman's rho correlation was used to examine the relationship between role limitations due to physical health problems and bodily pain. No significant correlation was found between role limitations due to physical health problems and bodily pain ($rho(72) = 0.030$, $p = 0.56$), suggesting that role limitations due to physical health problems are not associated with bodily pain.

Box 7.5 Point to consider

Calculating the Spearman's rho correlation by hand

The aim of this calculation is to simulate a study to examine whether there is a significant positive association between frequency of exercise (1 = Never, 2 = Monthly, 3 = Weekly, 4 = Every few days, 5 = Daily) and a self-report of physical health (1 = Very poor, 2 = Poor, 3 = OK, 4 = Good, 5 = Very good) among seven respondents.

Respondent	Frequency of exercise	Physical health	Rank frequency of exercise (Step 1)	Rank physical health (Step 1)	Difference (Step 2)	Difference squared (Step 3)
1	2	1	2.5	1	1.5	2.25
2	1	3	1	4.5	−3.5	12.25
3	3	2	4.5	2.5	2.0	4
4	4	4	6	5.5	0.5	0.25
5	5	4	7	5.5	1.5	2.25
6	3	2	4.5	2.5	2	4
7	2	3	2.5	4.5	−2	4

Step 1. Rank the scores for frequency of exercise and physical health in separate columns. If two people have exactly the same ranks, e.g. respondents 1 and 7 have the same score for frequency of exercise, then add ranks 2 + 3 (these would be ranked second and third) = 5, and divide by number of respondents, 2. Thus, 5/2 = 2.5.

Step 2. Subtract rank physical health from the ranks of frequency of exercise:

Respondent 1:   2.5 − 1 = 1.5

Respondent 2:   1 − 4.5 = −3.5

Respondent 3:   4.5 − 2.5 = 2

Respondent 4:   6 − 5.5 = 0.5

Respondent 5:   7 − 5.5 = 1.5

Respondent 6:   4.5 − 2.5 = 2

Respondent 7:   2.5 − 4.5 = −2

Step 3. Square each of the findings for step 2:

Respondent 1:   1.5 × 1.5 = 2.25

Respondent 2:   −3.5 × −3.5 = 12.25

Respondent 3:   2 × 2 = 4

Respondent 4:   0.5 × 0.5 = 0.25

Respondent 5:   1.5 × 1.5 = 2.25

Respondent 6:   2 × 2 = 4

Respondent 7:   −2 × −2 = 4

Step 4. Add together the results of step 3:

2.25 + 12.25 + 4 + 0.25 + 2.25 + 4 + 4 = 29.5

Step 5. Multiply the findings of step 4 by 6:

29.5 × 6 = 177

Step 6. Square the number of people in the sample and then minus 1:

(7 × 7) − 1 = 49 − 1 = 48

Step 7. Multiply the number of people in the sample by your finding for step 6:

7 × 48 = 336

Step 8. Divide your finding for step 5 by your finding for step 7:

177/336 = 0.5268

Step 9. Subtract your finding for step 8 from 1 to given you your Spearman's rho statistic:

1 − 0.5268 = 0.4732 = *rho*

Step 10. Subtract 2 from your sample size, *N* = 7, to give you your degrees of freedom:

d.f. = 7 − 2 = 5

Step 11. Look at the table and determine the number that accompanies the two-tailed test (we have made no particular statement regarding the direction of the relation between the two variables) for d.f. = 5 and a criterion level of 0.05. This number is 1.000. Our Spearman's rho (*rho* = 0.4732) is not larger than 1.000. Therefore, our finding is not significant and no significant correlation occurs between frequency of exercise and self-reported physical health.

	Significance levels for one-tailed test			
	0.05	0.025	0.01	0.005
	Significance levels for two-tailed test			
d.f.	0.10	0.05	0.02	0.01
5	0.900	1.000	1.000	
6	0.829	0.886	0.943	1.000
7	0.714	0.786	0.893	0.929
8	0.643	0.738	0.833	0.881

Some further things to know about correlations

So there we are. That is how you perform correlations. However, before we finish we just need to tell you three things about correlations. These are particularly useful things to consider when you are discussing your findings:

- correlation does not represent causation;
- issues of association;
- size of correlation.

Correlation does not represent causation

It is important to remember, when reporting any sort of correlation, not to infer that one variable *causes* another. Therefore, in the example above we could not conclude that role limitations due to physical health problems necessarily cause bodily pain, as it may be that worse body pain causes role limitations due to physical health problems. It is more likely that the two variables influence each other and/or work together. Remember to reflect this in your wording and always to talk about relationships, associations or correlations between two variables. Do not say that one variable causes another, unless you have a very good reason for thinking so.

Association

You will often find authors reporting the association between the two variables in a Pearson product-moment correlation coefficient, and this is thought to represent the shared variance between two variables. In theory, two variables can share a maximum of 100 per cent of the variance (identical) and a minimum of 0 per cent of variance (not related at all), and the association can be used to indicate the importance of a statistically significant relationship between two variables. The association is found by squaring (multiplying by itself) the r value, and reporting it as a percentage. In the example above, the correlation between role limitations due to physical health problems and bodily pain is 0.356. Therefore, to work out the association, calculate $0.356 \times 0.356 = 0.126736$, and report it as a percentage by multiplying the number by 100, so 12.6736 per cent, or 12.67 per cent (to two decimal places). You often find researchers reporting the variance as part of their discussion, sometimes used as an indicator of importance of the findings (or lack of importance of findings – as the smaller the percentage, the less important any relationship between the two variables).

Effect size: size of the correlation

The consideration of the importance of findings is now common practice in statistics. This importance of findings has become what is known as **effect size**. The consideration of effect size is an important addition to statistical testing through significance. Why? Well, significance levels depend on sample size. The larger the sample size, the lower the criterion is for finding a statistically significant result. For example, while a correlation of 0.2 is not statistically significant among a sample of 50 participants, a correlation of 0.2 will be statistically significant among a sample of 1,000 participants.

This has led to an interesting dilemma for researchers. Imagine two drug trials, one with drug A and one with drug B, both designed to help one particular illness.

- In the trial with drug A, among 50 participants, the correlation between drug A and improvement with patients was $r = 0.32$. The probability value was $p = 0.10$, not a statistically significant result.

- In the trial with drug B, among 1,000 participants, the correlation between drug B and improvement with patients was $r = 0.22$. The probability value was $p = 0.01$, a statistically significant result (though the correlation statistic is smaller than in the first study).

Therefore, if we studied these two drug trials separately we would come to different conclusions about the relationship between the two drugs and patient improvement. We would, based on significance testing, be likely to recommend drug B because there was statistically significant relationship between the drug and patient improvement, even though drug A had a stronger association with patient improvement.

This has led to a general rethink about reporting statistics, and the notion of considering effect size when reporting statistics. Effect size just refers to the strength of the relationship, and you will now commonly find a reference to the effect size of any finding in the literature.

Luckily, the criteria introduced by American statistician Jacob Cohen (1988) to label the effect size are used across the majority of the statistics mentioned (though it won't surprise you that practice varies, but to a lesser extent than in other areas of statistics). Cohen suggested that effect sizes of 0.2 to 0.5 should be regarded as 'small', 0.5 to 0.8 as 'moderate' and those above 0.8 as 'large'. Even luckier for us at this stage, when it comes to correlation statistics the r value is considered the indicator of effect size. So correlation statistics of:

- 0.2 represent a *small* effect size;
- 0.5 represent a *medium* (or *moderate*) effect size;
- 0.8 represent a *large* effect size.

It is best to see these criteria as set out in Table 7.1.

Remember, these are used as indicators of your findings to help you in your consideration. If you have a statistically significant correlation of 0.25, it is important not to conclude that this is a strong relationship. More importantly, if you have found a number of statistically significant correlations in your study, Cohen's criteria can be used to determine which correlations represent more important findings, and which are less important.

Let us consider effect size with some data in the adult dataset. Table 7.2 sets out the correlation between three variables: (1) the age of the respondents, (2) the number of falls they've had and (3) the number of other reported accidents.

Table 7.1 Cohen's effect size criteria

Criteria	Effect size
↑	1.0
	0.9
Large	0.8
↑	0.7
	0.6
Medium/moderate	0.5
	0.4
↑	0.3
Small	0.2
	0.1
	0.0

Table 7.2 Correlation coefficients between age of respondent, the number of falls they've had and the number of other accidents (apart from falls)

		Age	Number of falls	Number of other accidents reported (apart from falls)
Age	Pearson correlation	1	0.613[a]	0.239[b]
	Sig. (2-tailed)		0.000	0.040
	N	74	74	74
Number of falls	Pearson correlation	0.613[a]	1	0.355[a]
	Sig. (2-tailed)	0.000		0.002
	N	74	74	74
Number of other accidents reported (apart from falls)	Pearson correlation	0.239[b]	0.355[a]	1
	Sig. (2-tailed)	0.040	0.002	
	N	74	74	74

[a] Correlation is significant at the 0.01 level (2-tailed).
[b] Correlation is significant at the 0.05 level (2-tailed).

We can see that, although there is a statistically significant positive correlation between age and the number of other reported accidents ($r = 0.239$, $p < 0.05$), this correlation would be considered small. A much more important correlation to consider is the statistically significant positive correlation between age and the number of falls ($r = 0.613$, $p < 0.01$). The effect size of this correlation is medium to large, and therefore in any writing-up of the results we would emphasise this finding over the other finding regarding other types of accident.

Box 7.6 Point to consider

One last consideration of small effect sizes

There is one point to consider from a nursing perspective of small effect sizes. Robert Rosenthal (1991) has pointed out that the importance of effect sizes may depend on the sort of question we are investigating. For example, finding a small correlation between emergency ward volume and time spent at patients' bedsides might suggest that there isn't an important effect on emergency ward volume and the amount of bedside care. However, when it comes to aspects such as medication, if there is a small effect size between a new drug and its ability to save lives suggesting that it saves 4 out of 100 lives, if we translated that figure to a population of 100,000, that would mean 4,000 lives and the finding is certainly an important one regardless of the effect size. Therefore, we might, in nursing, have to consider what we are studying before drawing final conclusions.

Summary

In this chapter you have learnt the rationale for, the procedure for and the interpretation of two statistical tests:

✔ Pearson product–moment correlation;

✔ Spearman's rho correlation.

In the next chapter, we are going to introduce you to the final set of tests. Where, in this chapter, the tests we studied emphasised looking for statistically significant relationships and associations between variables, the next set of tests emphasises looking for *differences* between variables.

Self-assessment exercise

Pick one of the datasets that most closely matches your branch of nursing. Load it up and answer the corresponding question.

Adult branch

Terry Hainsworth (2004) reports the role of exercise is *important* in preventing falls among older patients. According to Hainsworth, falls are a major cause of disability and the leading cause of mortality due to injury in people over 75 in the UK. Therefore, Hainsworth finds that exercise might be encouraged in older people to prevent falls.

Does Hainsworth's observation apply to our current sample? What is the relationship between frequency of exercise (**freqexer**) and the numbers of falls people have had (**numberfalls**) among the current sample?

Remember to consider the skewness statistics for both variables to help you determine whether you should perform a Pearson or a Spearman correlation. Also consider the *r* or *rho* value, the direction of the relationship, whether it is significant and the effect size.

Mental health branch

In 2005, the *Nursing Times* published an article on insomnia (*Nursing Times*, 2005). The article suggests that insomnia could be classified into three areas: difficulty in falling asleep, early-morning awakening and difficulty in maintaining sleep. The article also refers to a number of factors that cause insomnia, including lifestyle factors such as alcohol and caffeine consumption, environmental factors such as noise and an uncomfortable bed, physical health problems, and psychological factors such as stress, depression and anxiety.

In the present study we have data on two of these variables, a self-rated variable on how difficult the person is finding it to stay asleep at night within the past week (difficultsleep) and the number of units of alcohol they have consumed during the last week (alcoholconsumption). Examine whether there is a statistically significant relationship between difficulty in staying asleep at night and the number of units of alcohol the person has consumed during the week.

Remember to consider the skewness statistics for both variables to help you determine whether you should perform a Pearson or a Spearman correlation. Also consider the *r* or *rho* value, the direction of the relationship, whether it is significant and the effect size.

Learning disability branch

Catherine Bernal (2005) discussed the maintenance of oral health in people with learning disabilities. She suggests that the oral health of individuals with learning disabilities is often threatened, as they are reliant upon their carers for the maintenance of their oral health.

In our sample, we have data that look at this issue, a first variable being an assessment by the disability nurse of the extent to which the person with the learning disability can adequately deal with their own oral hygiene (**oralhygcapability**), and the number of fillings or extensive dental work the person has had in the past three years (**amountofdentalwork**). Examine whether there is a statistically significant relationship between the extent to which the person with the learning disability can adequately deal with their own oral hygiene and the number of fillings or extensive dental work the person has had in the past three years.

Remember to consider the skewness statistics for both variables to help you determine whether you should perform a Pearson or a Spearman correlation. Also consider the *r* or *rho* value, the direction of the relationship, whether it is significant and the effect size.

Child branch

Helena Dunbar (2001) looked at improving the management of asthma in under-fives. One of the things that Dunbar notes is that children who wheeze can be divided into two groups: those who wheeze for a very short time and those who wheeze persistently and go on to develop asthma. Dunbar suggests that one way to assess the difference between asthma and wheezing is to monitor different symptoms, including recurrent or persistent night-time waking.

In our dataset we can explore these ideas by looking at the relationship between two variables: a parental assessment of both the percentage of time they feel their child spends wheezing (**wheezing**) and the percentage of time where there is recurrent or persistent night-time waking (**waking**).

Remember to consider the skewness statistics for both variables to help you determine whether you should perform a Pearson or a Spearman correlation. Also consider the *r* or *rho* value, the direction of the relationship, whether it is significant and the effect size.

Further reading

We would encourage you to read the articles mentioned in the self-assessment section to develop ideas around these topics. They are all available free online (on registering) at the *Nursing Times* website: http://www.nursingtimes.net/. The references for the articles are:

Bernal, C. (2005) 'Maintenance of oral health in people with learning disabilities', *Nursing Times*, 101(6): 40–42.

Dunbar, H. (2001) 'Improving the management of asthma in under-fives', *Nursing Times*, 97(31): 36.

Hainsworth, T. (2004) 'The role of exercise in falls prevention for older patients', *Nursing Times*, 100(18): 28–29.

Nursing Times (2005) 'Insomnia', 101(39): 25.

You will be able to access the articles by typing the first author's surname or the title of the paper in the Search box on the website.

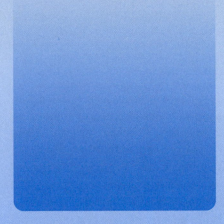

Chapter 8

Comparing average scores: statistics for all sorts of groups and occasions

Key themes

- Mean scores
- Independent-samples *t*-test
- Paired-samples *t*-test
- Wilcoxon sign-ranks test
- Mann–Whitney *U* test

Learning outcomes

By the end of this chapter you will learn the rationale for, the procedure for and the interpretation in SPSS for Windows of the following four inferential statistical tests:

- Independent-samples *t*-test
- Paired-samples *t*-test
- Wilcoxon sign-ranks test
- Mann–Whitney *U* test

Introduction

Imagine . . . That you are a learning disability nurse and have been working with carers for people with learning disabilities. Your work has been primarily focused on tending to the needs of these carers because, if these carers become burned out and stressed at work, the level of support that they can provide to their clients will be adversely affected. You are conducting a study to see how you can reduce the amount of work-related stress among this type of carer group. From a preliminary survey of a sample of these carers, it looks as if they would benefit from a support group which would enable them to mutually support each other in an informal and systematic way. You have decided to measure the carers' work stress levels before introducing a support group scheme so that you can see how stressed they are before and afterwards. By means of a statistical test, you would be able to see whether the support group scheme is working. On the other hand, you might want to compare participants in the support group scheme with those who haven't yet been able to take part (that is, a control group). Are there significant differences in the work stress levels of participants versus non-participants? We will look at the case of the work stress of carers for people with learning disabilities later in the chapter.

In the previous chapter we looked at correlation statistics, which are statistics that find out whether there is a relationship between two continuous-type variables (such as age and wage earning). However, there are other statistics that are used for measuring variables before and after an intervention (such as the support group scheme for carers) or for assessing group differences in a variable (for example, comparing participants in the support group scheme with non-participants).

In this chapter we are going to look at these tests. You are going to use again terms such as significance testing and scores, but you will also learn the rationale for, the procedure for and the interpretation of four new statistical tests. As you can see from Figure 8.1, the four tests are:

- Two parametric tests:
  - **Independent-samples *t*-test** – used when you have one categorical-type variable with two levels, and one continuous-type variable that you have decided can be used in a parametric test.
  - **Paired-samples *t*-test** – used when you have the *same* continuous-type variable, administered on two occasions, and you have decided the data are suitable for use in a parametric test.
- Non-parametric tests:
  - **Mann–Whitney *U* test** – used when you have one categorical-type variable with two levels, and one continuous-type variable that you have decided to use in a non-parametric test.

Question 1 What combination of variables do you have?	Which statistical test to use	Question 2 Should your continuous-type data be used with parametric tests or non-parametric tests?	Which statistical test to use
Two continuous-type variables, which is the same variable administered twice	Go to question 2	Parametric Non-parametric	Paired-samples *t*-test Wilcoxon sign-ranks test
One categorical-type and one continuous-type variable	Go to question 2	Parametric Non-parametric	Independent-samples *t*-test Mann-Whitney *U* test

Figure 8.1 Part of the decision-making table (Figure 6.6) that relates to statistical tests that compare groups and occasions

● **Wilcoxon sign-ranks test** – used when the *same* continuous-type variable has been administered on two occasions but you have decided to use the variables in a non-parametric test.

Energiser

Before you start we are going to get your brain warmed up mathematically, and get you to carry out some simple calculations (in your head). Although these calculations may seem rather simple and redundant, the tasks are related to some of the concepts you will come across in the chapter and will help your understanding. If you can do these, then you are well on your way to understanding the statistics covered in this chapter.

1. Which is the highest of these five numbers?

    7.87   7.32   7.52   7.23   7.93

2. Which is the lowest of these five numbers?

    4.27   2.92   3.52   2.83   3.33

3. Subtract 7.56 from 13.23.

4. Subtract 13.23 from 7.56.

5. Subtract 234.33 from 432.21.

6. Subtract 543.94 from 329.06.

Comparing differences

The common theme among these four tests is that they compare the average scores of variables (average scores are covered in Chapter 3) across certain occasions. The four tests can be first put into two categories (aside from being parametric and non-parametric), as follows.

● Group 1: tests that compare two groups of subjects on a continuous-type variable (independent groups)

In the title of this chapter we referred to tests that can be used to compare groups of data. These tests compare two groups of data on a continuous-type variable. A simple example of this would be male and female nurses (these are two groups: male nurses and female nurses) might be compared on their average wages to find out whether there are equal pay structures in the profession.

An example from the research literature of the way this type of test is used is provided in the study by Maureen Smith (2005). Smith wanted to examine whether encouragement and praise during an eye acuity test (a test for sharpness and clearness of eyesight) improved patients' performance. Therefore, she compared two groups of people who underwent eye examinations: one group received encouragement from the nurse (for example, 'Well done' and 'That was good, see if you can read any further') and the other group received no such encouragement. A group 1 type of t-test would be used to compare the two groups on how well they did on the eye acuity test, with the expectation that the 'encouragement' group would have done better.

The two tests that fall into this group are:

● the independent-samples t-test - this is the parametric version within this group of tests;

● the Mann–Whitney U test - this is a non-parametric version within this group of tests.

(Remember the differences between parametric and non-parametric are to do with the normal distribution. To read more on the other issues and issues of skewness go back to Chapter 6.)

A term that is used to sum up these types of tests is that they are tests dealing with **independent groups/samples** of data. In other words, whether your continuous variable is parametric or non-parametric, you, as researcher in this situation, are comparing two *independent* (or unrelated) groups of cases on the same variable (in our example, people who were encouraged by the nurse in the eye acuity tests and those that were not encouraged by the nurse in the eye acuity tests).

● Group 2: tests that compare the same subjects on a continuous-type variable on two occasions (dependent groups)

In the title of this chapter we referred to tests that can be used to compare data on two occasions. These tests compare two sets of data on the same continuous variable on two separate occasions. A simple example of this would be comparing average patients' ratings of pain (scored on a scale of 1 = No pain at all to 10 = A lot of pain) before and after taking a new drug designed to decrease pain.

An example from the research literature, where this test might be used, was demonstrated by Christopher Hodgkins and his colleagues (Hodgkins *et al.*, 2005). Stress has been identified as an important issue among residential carers looking after individuals with learning disabilities. Staff were asked by Hodgkins and his co-workers to assess themselves on a measure of stress. The staff then underwent an intervention programme according to their needs in which it was ensured that they had support, such as appropriate training, regular staff meetings, reviews of internal procedures, and guidance in counselling skills and how to respond to stressful situations. Three months later, staff assessed themselves again on the same measure of stress. This type of *t*-test would be used to compare the two occasions in term of people's scores, with the expectation that stress would be lower after the three-month period.

The two tests that fall into this group are:

- the paired-sample *t*-test – this is the parametric version within this group of tests;
- the Wilcoxon sign-ranks test – this is the non-parametric version within this group of tests.

A term that is used to sum up these types of tests is that they are tests that are dealing with **dependent groups** of data. In other words, whether your continuous variable is parametric or non-parametric, you, as researcher in this situation, are comparing two dependent (or related) groups of cases on the same variable (in our example, the same group of carers *before* and *after* a clinical intervention).

Comparing groups: tests that compare groups of subjects on a continuous-type variable

In this section we are going to introduce you to two tests: the independent-samples *t*-test and the Mann–Whitney *U* test. These two tests are very similar in nature and are used to see whether there are statistically significant differences between two levels of a categorical variable on a continuous variable. The major difference between these two tests is that the independent-samples *t*-test is used when the continuous variable comprises parametric data and the Mann–Whitney *U* test is used when the continuous variable comprises non-parametric data.

Box 8.1 Point to consider

Different names for the same independent-samples *t*-test

The independent-samples *t*-test is known by a number of names. These include unmatched *t*-test, *t*-test for two independent means, independent *t*-test, *t*-test for unrelated samples, and Student's *t*-test. Do not concern yourself; they all refer to the same test.

Comparing groups, test number 1: independent-samples *t*-test (parametric test)

The independent-samples *t*-test (see also Box 8.1) is used to compare mean scores for a continuous-type variable (that you want to treat as usable in a parametric test) across two levels of a categorical-type variable.

To explain this simply and fully, let us use an example from one of the datasets, the learning disability dataset. In this dataset there are 20 questions relating to 24 people diagnosed as having learning difficulties. Two of the questions in this dataset refer to the sex of the person with the learning disability and the number of consultations the person has had with the learning disability nurse. Say, for example, we are interested in whether there is a sex difference in patients in terms of the number of times they have visited the nurse. Here, sex of the person is categorical, whereas the number of visits is continuous. What the independent-samples *t*-test allows the researcher to do is to compare the number of visits to the learning disability nurse made by the two groups of people and determine whether there is a *difference* between males and females in their number of consultations.

What the independent-samples *t*-test does is work out for each group the mean score on the continuous variable (visits) by each group and then calculate whether there is a difference between the group, by means of the *t* statistic (which looks at the scores, and the spread of scores) and significance testing (that is, working out whether any differences observed between the groups are not likely to have occurred by chance and we can be confident of our results).

Therefore, what the statistical test will do, in our case, is work out the mean number of visits for males and the mean number of visits for females, and then use a statistical test to decide whether the difference between the two values found is statistically significant.

Table 8.1 Actual number of consultations with the learning-disability nurse by sex, and mean number of consultations by sex

Males (*N* = 14)	Females (*N* = 10)
10	18
28	5
4	12
8	13
12	3
25	5
8	6
10	2
12	7
7	3
2	
14	
16	
16	
Mean = total of scores (172) divided by number of cases (14) Mean number of consultations = 12.29	Mean = total of scores (64) divided by number of cases (10) Mean number of consultations = 6.40

Table 8.1 shows the first part of this operation, a table of all the scores in the dataset by each group (males and females), and the mean score for each of these groups.

On the face of it, on average, male patients have had more consultations with the learning disability nurse more times than females. However, remember that because this is a sample we are never 100 per cent confident of any relationships or differences we observe with descriptive statistics, and therefore we need to test whether there is a statistically significant difference. What is crucial with the independent-samples *t*-test is that it allows you to determine whether there is a statistically significant difference *between* groups of respondents in their number of visits to the learning disability nurse.

To find this out, let us carry out this test with these data on SPSS for Windows.

Independent-samples t-test using SPSS for Windows

To perform the Independent-samples *t*-test using SPSS for Windows, click on the **Analyze** pull-down menu and click on **Compare Means**, then click on **Independent-Samples t Test**. You will then get a screen that looks similar to that in Figure 8.2 (however, on your screen the **Test Variable(s):** and the **Grouping Variable:** boxes should be blank).

Highlight the variable **Number of Consultations [consulta]** in the left-hand box and move it into the **Test Variables(s):** box by clicking on the arrow button. Similarly, highlight the grouping variable **sex** and transfer it to the **Grouping Variable:** box. At this

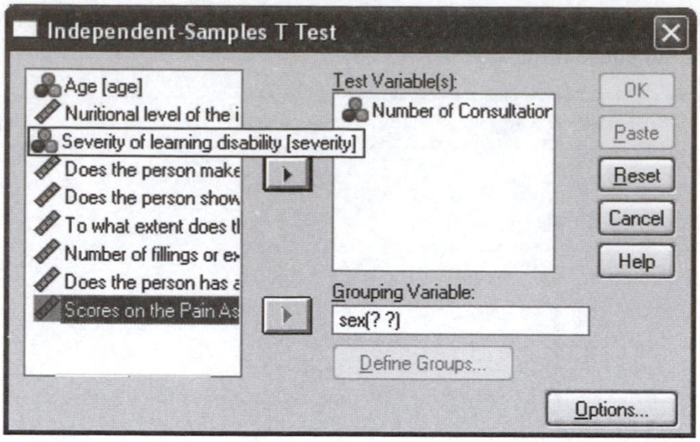

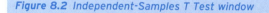

Figure 8.2 *Independent-Samples T Test window*

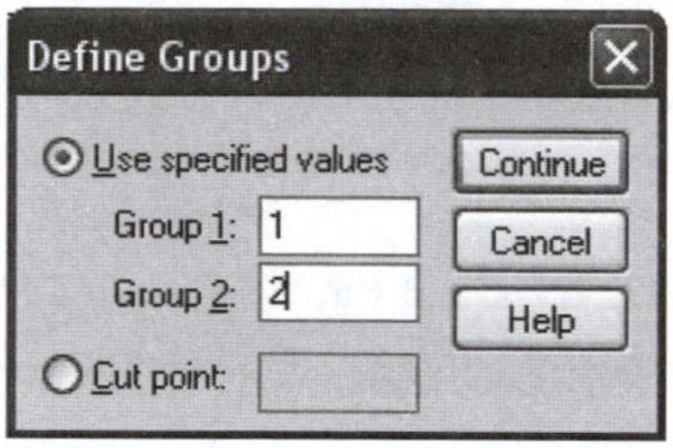

Figure 8.3 *Define Groups window*

point the **Grouping Variable:** box will appear with **[? ?]**. You now have to assign the values of the categorical variable by clicking on **Define Groups** (Figure 8.3). Now type the values of our categorical variable into the boxes. For sex, the values are 1 for males and 2 for females. Type the value **1** into the **Group 1:** box and type 2 into the **Group 2:** box, then click on **Continue**. The values 1, 2 will appear in the brackets after **sex**.

Now click on **OK** to run the *t*-test. Your output should look like that in Figure 8.4.

In this output we have all the information we need to interpret whether a statistically significant difference occurs between males and females in terms of the number of consultations they have made to the learning disability nurse. As usual, we will use the 'describe and decide' rule introduced previously to reach our conclusions about the data.

Using 'describe and decide' to interpret the independent-samples t-test

From the output in Figure 8.4, you will need to consider three things:

Group Statistics

	Sex of patient	N	Mean	Std. Deviation	Std. Error Mean
Number of Consultations with learning disability nurse	Male	14	12.29	7.279	1.945
	Female	10	6.40	3.718	1.176

> Means and standard deviations for males and females

Independent Samples Test

		Levene's Test for Equality of Variances		t-test for Equality of Means						
									95% Confidence Interval of the Difference	
		F	Sig.	t	df	Sig. (2-tailed)	Mean Difference	Std. Error Difference	Lower	Upper
Number of Consultations with learning disability nurse	Equal variances assumed	2.428	.133	2.338	22	.029	5.886	2.517	.665	11.106
	Equal variances not assumed			2.589	20.315	.017	5.886	2.273	1.149	10.623

> *t* value

> Sig. 2-tailed

Figure 8.4 *Independent-samples* t*-test output for comparing males and females on their number of consultations with the learning disability nurse*

- *Mean scores and standard deviations*. These are the basis of our description. We note both the mean scores (with the standard deviation, which is a statistic that indicates the spread of scores) and which mean score is higher.

- *The* t *value*. The statistical test statistic. Unlike the Pearson product-moment correlation in Chapter 7, it is not important to note whether the statistic is positive or minus. You will notice that you are provided with two *t* statistics. Read the **Equal Variances assumed** line, because you are using a parametric test and, therefore, you have assumed you are using continuous data that fulfil this criterion. There is more information on this in Box 8.2.

- The *Sig. (2-tailed)*. The significance level. This is the probability level given to the current findings. The significance level found in the bullet point above tells the researcher whether the difference noted between the means is significant. Remember, if this figure is below the $p = 0.05$ or $p = 0.01$ criterion then the finding is statistically significant. If this figure is above 0.05 then the findings are not statistically significant.

Therefore, the average mean score for males in terms of their number of consultations with the learning disability nurse is 12.29 (with a standard deviation of 7.279, though in writing it up we abbreviate this figure to one decimal place: 7.3). This means that, on average, males have around 12 consultations with the learning disability nurse. The mean score for females in terms of their number of consultations with the learning disability nurse is 6.40 (with a standard deviation of 3.71, which we abbreviate to one decimal place: 3.7). This means that, on average, females have around six consultations

Box 8.2 Point to consider

Levene's test for equality of variance

You remember some of the other rules in Chapter 6 about data being suitable for use in parametric tests. One was if two continuous-type variables are being used or compared, then they must have similar standard deviations. We told you then not to worry too much about some of these aspects, and Levene's test for equality of variance is one reason for this. Levene's test for equality of variance gives you the option to use an independent-samples t-test even when your standard deviations (variances) are not similar. (This sort of statistic is known as a correction statistic, because you are seeking to correct possible errors.)

You will see in the lower table of Figure 8.4 the statistics for Levene's test for equality of variances, with the test statistic (F) and then the significance (Sig.) value. If this significance value is greater than 0.05, then you can assume equal variances. If this happens, as it has in our example, it is recommended that you just ignore this statistic.

However, if it is significant, do not worry. Just read the **Equal variances not assumed** line. You are also recommended to report this when you write up your analysis. If you do this you need to include a simple line such as 'Levene's test for equality of variance suggested that equal variances could not be assumed (F = test statistic, $p < 0.05$), and therefore t was corrected for equal variances not assumed.'

with the learning disability nurse. Therefore, we would observe that males have more consultations with the learning disability nurse than females.

Next is the t value. The t value for the independent-samples t-test is 2.338. This tells us very little at this stage. However, the significance level is $p = 0.029$. This is smaller than 0.05. Therefore, we conclude that there *is* a statistically significant difference between males and females for the number of consultations with the learning disability nurse. This finding suggests that males have statistically significantly more consultations with the learning disability nurse than do females.

Using 'describe and decide' to report the independent-samples t-test

The next stage is to report these statistics. There is a formal way of reporting the independent-samples t-test, which comprises two elements. First there is a formal statement of your statistics, which must include the following:

- *The test statistic.* Each test has a symbol for its statistic. The independent-samples *t*-test uses the symbol *t*. Your write-up must include what *t* is equal to. In the example above, $t = 2.338$; however, we would abbreviate this to two decimals places, therefore $t = 2.34$.

- *The degrees of freedom.* This concept was introduced in Chapter 6, and is traditionally reported (though it is worth noting that it is not always reported). For the independent-samples *t*-test, the degrees of freedom equal the size of your sample minus 2. Here, the minus 2 represents minus 1 for each sample, because you have asked only two sets of respondents (males and females). The figure is placed between the *t* and the equals sign and is written in brackets. Here the degrees of freedom are 22 (size of sample = 24, minus 2 = 22). Therefore, $t(22) = 2.34$.

- *The probability.* Remember that there are two ways to report the probability:

  - The traditional way is to report whether your probability value is below 0.05 or 0.01 (statistically significant) or above 0.05 (not statistically significant). Here, you use less than (<) or greater than (>) the criteria levels. You state these criteria by reporting whether $p < 0.05$ (statistically significant), $p < 0.01$ (statistically significant) or $p > 0.05$ (not statistically significant). So in the example above, as $p = 0.029$, we would write $p < 0.05$ and place this after the reporting of the *t* value. Therefore, with our findings, $t(22) = 2.34, p < 0.05$.

  - More recently, statisticians and researchers have started reporting the *p* value as it is; in our case, $p = 0.029$. Therefore, in the present case, we would write $t(22) = 2.34, p = 0.029$. It is important to note that practice varies, and your lecturers may insist on using the more traditional method, but today most disciplines suggest writing *p* as its actual value. What is important to note is that you still interpret the statistical significance of your findings in terms of its being greater or less than 0.05 and 0.01; it's just that you report the actual probability value rather than use the < and > signs.

This must then be incorporated into the text, to help the reader understand and conceptualise your findings. In writing the text use the 'describe and decide' rule to inform the reader of your finding:

- remind the reader of the two variables you are examining;
- say which mean score is the higher;
- tell the reader whether the finding is statistically significant or not.

You can use all the information above to write a fairly simple sentence which conveys your findings succinctly but effectively. Therefore, using the findings above we might report:

An independent-samples *t*-test was used to examine statistically significant differences between males and females in terms of the number of consultations they had

Box 8.3 Point to consider

Writing up a non-significant result for independent-samples *t*-test: an example

An independent-samples *t*-test was used to examine differences between males and females in terms of the number of consultations they had with the learning disability nurse. No significant difference ($t(22) = 0.21$, $p = 0.23$ ($p > 0.05$)) was found between females (mean = 7.34, S.D. = 7.0) and males (mean = 7.84, S.D. = 7.3) in terms of the number of consultations they had with the learning disability nurse. This suggests that there are no sex differences in the number of consultations people have with the learning disability nurse.

with the learning disability nurse. Males (mean = 12.29, S.D. = 7.3) scored statistically significantly higher ($t(22) = 2.34$, $p = 0.029$) than females (mean = 6.40, S.D. = 3.7) in terms of their number of consultations with the learning disability nurse. This finding suggests that males have statistically significantly more consultations with the learning disability nurse than do females.

Again, you will come across different ways of writing up tests, but you will find all the information included above in any write-up. Read Boxes 8.3–8.5 for further points to consider when using an independent-samples *t*-test.

● Comparing groups, test number 2: Mann–Whitney *U* test (non-parametric test)

If you have got to grips with the independent-samples *t*-test, then the good news is that all the three remaining tests are variations on this theme of seeing whether there is a statistically significant difference between two sets of scores. The first of these is the Mann–Whitney *U* test.

The Mann–Whitney *U* test is the non-parametric alternative to the independent-samples *t*-test. The independent-sample *t*-test is used to examine for a statistically significant difference between two levels of a categorical variable on a continuous variable that is described as parametric data. The Mann–Whitney *U* test is used to examine for statistically significant differences between two levels of a categorical variable on a continuous variable that is described as *non-parametric* data.

Performing the Mann–Whitney U test in SPSS for Windows

To illustrate the Mann–Whitney *U* test we are going to look at the child branch dataset. In this dataset, 40 mothers have been asked about their attitudes towards immunisation

Box 8.4 Point to consider

Comparing groups when you have more than two levels

Sometimes you might want to compare two groups of a variable but you have more than two levels of the categorical variable. For example, in the adult branch dataset there is a variable **care** which describes the type of care the person is receiving at the moment:

1 = Person at home (alone)

2 = Person at home (with a carer who is a relative)

3 = Person at home (with a carer who is not a relative)

4 = Person in a nursing home

5 = Person in a hospital

Say, for example, you want to compare people in a nursing home (group 4 above) and people in a hospital (group 5) on a continuous variable for mobility of the person. All you need do in the independent-samples *t*-test procedure on SPSS is to insert the number of the two groups you wish to compare, in this case 4 and 5.

Define Groups

- ⦿ Use specified values

  Group 1: 4

  Group 2: 5

- ◯ Cut point:

  Continue

  Cancel

  Help

Box 8.5 Point to consider

Calculation of independent-samples *t*-test by hand

Self-rated mobility scores are compared by males and females, to see whether there are sex differences in mobility. To make it easy for calculations, ratings of mobility range from 1 (not at all mobile) to 5 (very mobile). The same scale was administered to five males and five females. The researcher doesn't make a prediction of whether women or men will score significantly higher.

	Men			Women	
	Mobility			Mobility	
1	4	16 (Step 1)	1	3	9 (Step 7)
2	5	25 (Step 1)	2	2	4 (Step 7)
3	5	25 (Step 1)	3	4	16 (Step 7)
4	2	4 (Step 1)	4	5	25 (Step 7)
5	3	9 (Step 1)	5	4	16 (Step 7)

First work out the mean and standard deviation for men and women for their scores on mobility as follows:

Step 1. Square each of the scores for men:

$4 \times 4 = 16$, $5 \times 5 = 25$, $5 \times 5 = 25$, $2 \times 2 = 4$, $3 \times 3 = 9$

Step 2. Add up all the scores for men:

$4 + 5 + 5 + 2 + 3 = 19$

Step 3. Add up all the scores obtained from step 1:

$16 + 25 + 25 + 4 + 9 = 79$

Step 4. Square the result of step 2:

$19 \times 19 = 361$

Step 5. Divide the result of step 4 by the number of men:

$361/5 = 72.2$

Step 6. Subtract the findings in step 5 from the result in step 3:

$79 - 72.2 = 6.8$

Step 7. Square each of the scores for women:

$3 \times 3 = 9$, $2 \times 2 = 4$, $4 \times 4 = 16$, $5 \times 5 = 25$, $4 \times 4 = 16$

Step 8. Add up all the scores for women:

$3 + 2 + 4 + 5 + 4 = 18$

Step 9. Add up all the scores obtained from step 7:

$9 + 4 + 16 + 25 + 16 = 70$

• • •

Step 10. Square the result of step 8:

$18 \times 18 = 324$

Step 11. Divide the result of step 10 by the number of women:

$324/5 = 64.8$

Step 12. Subtract the findings in step 11 from the result in step 9:

$70 - 64.8 = 5.2$

Step 13. Add the results of step 6 and step 12:

$6.8 + 5.2 = 12$

Step 14. Add the number of men to the number of women and then subtract 2. This gives you your degrees of freedom:

d.f. $= 5 + 5 - 2 = 8$

Step 15. Add the number of men to the number of women:

$5 + 5 = 10$

Step 16. Multiply the number of men by the number of women:

$5 \times 5 = 25$

Step 17. Divide the findings of step 15 by the findings of step 16:

$10/25 = 0.4$

Step 18. Divide the result of step 13 by the finding of step 14:

$12/(10 - 2) \ldots 12/8 = 1.5$

Step 19. Multiply the result of step 18 by the finding of step 17:

$1.5 \times 0.4 = 0.6$

Step 20. Find the square root of step 19:

$\sqrt{0.6} = 0.7746$

Step 21. Work out the mobilty mean score for men:

$19/5 = 3.8$

Step 22. Work out the mobilty mean score for women:

$18/5 = 3.6$

▶

Step 23. Subtract the result of step 22 from the result of step 21:

$3.8 - 3.6 = 0.2$

Step 24. Divide the result of step 23 by the finding in step 20. This will give you your t value:

$t = 0.2/0.7746 = 0.2581$

Use the table below to determine the significance of your result.

	Significance levels for two-tailed test			
	0.05	0.025	0.01	0.0005
	Significance levels for one-tailed test			
d.f.	0.10	0.05	0.02	0.01
6	1.943	2.447	3.143	3.707
7	1.895	2.365	2.998	3.499
8	1.860	2.306	2.896	3.355
9	1.833	2.262	2.821	3.250
10	1.812	2.228	2.764	3.169

Degrees of freedom were calculated in step 14 (d.f. = 8).

We will use a two-tailed test (as there is no prediction which sex will score higher on mobility) and we will also use a significance level of 0.05. The value for degrees of freedom = 8, two-tailed test and a significance level of 0.05 is 1.860. Our t is 0.2581 which is smaller than the value quoted in the table. Therefore we would conclude that there is no significant difference in mobility between men and women.

of their child against measles, mumps and rubella by means of the MMR jab. We will look at the relationship between two variables: whether the child is their first child and their response to the statement 'I can protect my child from exposure to measles, mumps and rubella without the MMR jab'. Responses are scored on a five-point scale to this question: 1 = Strongly disagree, 2 = Disagree, 3 = Undecided, 4 = Agree and 5 = Strongly agree. Therefore, someone scoring highest on this variable thinks they can protect their child from measles, mumps or rubella without the MMR jab.

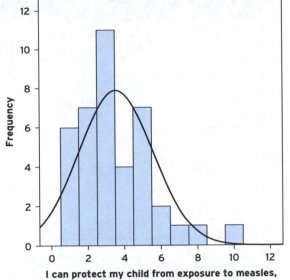

	N	Minimum	Maximum	Mean	Std.	Skewness	
	Statistic	Statistic	Statistic	Statistic	Statistic	Statistic	Std. Error
I can protect my child from exposure to measles, mumps and rubella without the MMR jab	40	1	10	3.53	2.025	1.083	.374
Valid N (listwise)	40						

Descriptive Statistics

Figure 8.5 *Histogram of responses to the statement 'I can protect my child from exposure to measles, mumps and rubella without the MMR jab'*

The first thing to show you is that the attitude towards the MMR jab might represent non-parametric data. Although different people take different attitudes towards whether numerical data should be treated as parametric or non-parametric, an examination of the distribution of the scores via a histogram (see Figure 8.5) suggests that the scores of this variable do not represent a normal distribution (see how the bars don't fit with the normal distribution shown by the black line), and the skewness statistics is above 1. Therefore, we should treat these continuous-type data as non-parametric.

To perform the Mann–Whitney *U* test click on the **Analyze** pull-down menu and click on **Nonparametric Tests**. Next click on **2 independent samples**. Highlight the continuous variable **I can protect my child from exposure . . . (protectMMR)** in the left-hand box and move it to the **Test Variable List** box by clicking on the arrow button (Figure 8.6).

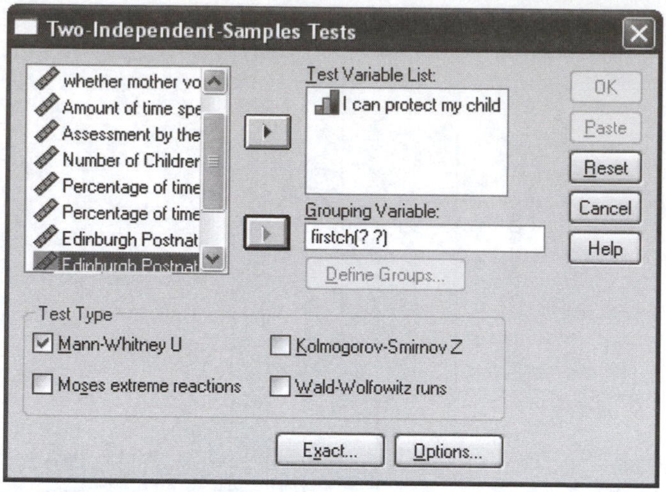

Figure 8.6 SPSS screen for the Mann–Whitney U test

Similarly, highlight the categorical variable (**Is s/he your first child [firstch]**) and transfer it to the **Grouping Variable:**. Define the values of the grouping (independent) variable by clicking on **Define Groups**, and clicking **0** (No) and **1** (Yes) into the boxes. Make sure that **Mann–Whitney *U*** is ticked in the **Test Type** box, then click **Continue**, then **OK** to get your output (see Figure 8.7).

In this output we have all the information we need to interpret whether a statistically significant difference occurs between mothers for whom this is their first child and mothers for whom this is not their first child in thinking they can protect their child from measles, mumps and rubella without the MMR jab. Again, remember to *describe* and then *decide*.

Using 'describe and decide' to interpret the Mann–Whitney U test

From the output in Figure 8.7, you will need to consider three things:

- *Mean ranks*. These are the basis of our description, and are used in a similar way to the mean scores for the independent-samples *t*-test. Here, lower ranks mean lower scores (remember 2, 5, 7, 10, 13 would be ranked 1, 2, 3, 4, 5). We note the mean ranks and then which mean rank is higher.

- *The* U *value*. The test statistic.

- *The Asymp Sig. (2-tailed)*. The significance level. This is the probability level given to the current findings. The significance level informs the researcher whether there are statistically significant differences between the means scores. Remember, if this figure is below the $p = 0.05$ or $p = 0.01$ criterion, then the finding is statistically significant. If this figure is above 0.05, then the findings are not statistically significant.

Ranks

	Is s/he your first child?	N	Mean Rank	Sum of Ranks
I can protect my child from exposure to measles, mumps and rubella without the MMR jab	No	20	16.55	331.00
	Yes	20	24.45	489.00
	Total	40		

Mean rank

Test Statistics[b]

	I can protect my child from exposure to measles, mumps and rubella without the MMR jab
Mann-Whitney U	121.000
Wilcoxon W	331.000
Z	-2.176
Asymp. Sig. (2-tailed)	.030
Exact Sig. [2*(1-tailed Sig.)]	.033[a]

U statistic

Significance level

a. Not corrected for ties.
b. Grouping Variable: Is s/he your first child?

Figure 8.7 SPSS output for Mann–Whitney U test for our example in comparing mothers on whether they believe they can protect their child from exposure to measles, mumps and rubella without the MMR jab in terms of whether it is their first child

In the present example, the mean rank for mothers for whom the child is their first child is 24.45. The mean rank for mothers for whom the child is not their first child is 16.55. In this case, it is mothers for whom the child is their firstborn who score higher on the variable.

The U value for the statistic is 121.00. This tells us very little at this stage. However, the significance level is $p = 0.030$. This is smaller than 0.05 and so we conclude that there is a statistically significant difference between the two sets of mothers in their belief they can protect their child from measles, mumps and rubella without the MMR jab. Therefore, the mean ranks suggest that mothers for whom the child is their first child tend to believe more than mothers for whom the child is not their first child that they can protect their child from measles, mumps and rubella without the MMR jab.

Using 'describe and decide' to report the Mann–Whitney U test

The next stage is to report these statistics. There is a formal way of reporting the Mann-Whitney U test, which comprises two elements. First there is a formal statement of your statistics, which must include the following:

- *The test statistic*. Each test has a symbol for its statistic. The Mann–Whitney U test has the symbol U. Therefore, in your write-up you must include what U is equal to. In the example, $U = 121.00$.

- *The probability*. Remember from the previous two chapters that there are two ways to report the probability:

  - The traditional way is to report whether your probability value is below 0.05 or 0.01 (statistically significant) or above 0.05 (not statistically significant). Here, you use less than (<) or greater than (>) the criteria levels. You state these criteria by reporting whether $p < 0.05$ (statistically significant), $p < 0.01$ (statistically significant) or $p > 0.05$ (not statistically significant). So, in the example above, as $p = 0.030$, we would write $p < 0.05$ and place this after the reporting of the U value. Therefore, with our findings, $U = 121$, $p < 0.05$.

  - More recently, statisticians and researchers have started reporting the p value as it is; in our case $p = 0.030$. Therefore, in the present case we would write $U = 121$, $p = 0.030$.

This must then be incorporated into the text, to help the reader understand and conceptualise your findings. In writing up the text use the 'describe and decide' rule to inform the reader of your finding:

- Remind the reader of the two variables you are examining.
- Say which mean score is the higher.
- Tell the reader whether the finding is statistically significant or not.

You can use all the information above to write a fairly simple sentence which conveys your findings succinctly but effectively. Therefore, using the findings above we might report:

A Mann–Whitney U test was used to examine statistically significant differences between mothers who had children who were their firstborn, and mothers for whom their child was not their firstborn, and their belief that they can protect their child from measles, mumps and rubella without the MMR jab. Mothers for whom the child was their firstborn (mean rank = 24.45) were found to score statistically significantly higher ($U = 121.00$, $p = 0.03$) than mothers for whom the child was not their first born (mean rank = 16.55). This finding suggests that mothers with children, for whom it is their first child, believe that they can protect their child from measles, mumps and rubella without the MMR jab more so than mothers with children, for whom it is not their first child.

Again, you will come across different ways of writing up tests, but you will find all the information included above in any write-up. However, if you want to expand your knowledge a little then read Boxes 8.6–8.8.

Box 8.6 Point to consider

Writing up a non-significant result for a Mann-Whitney *U* test: an example

A Mann–Whitney *U* test was used to examine significant differences between mothers who had children for whom it was their firstborn, and mothers who had children for whom it was not their firstborn, and their belief that they can protect their child from measles, mumps and rubella without the MMR jab. No significant difference was found for their belief in protecting their child ($U = 0.50$, $p = 0.73$ [or $p > 0.05$]) was found between mothers for whom the child was a firstborn (mean rank = 9.31) and mothers for whom the child was not a firstborn (mean rank = 9.23).

Box 8.7 Point to consider

Medians rather than mean ranks for the Mann-Whitney *U* test

It doesn't quite end here with the Mann–Whitney *U* test. Unlike its parametric counterpart, the Independent-samples *t*-test, which reports the mean and standard deviations, here the descriptive statistics include mean ranks, which aren't as familiar or as informative to people. Therefore, some people prefer to give the median score along with the semi-interquartile range as an indicator of variability, as this is more informative. (We outlined the median and the semi-interquartile range in Chapter 3.) It is a temptation not to give the median score when performing the Mann–Whitney *U* test as SPSS for Windows does not give you median scores when it prints out the Mann–Whitney *U* test statistics. Nonetheless, we would recommend that you consider providing this medium and the semi-interquartile range instead of the mean rank scores as these are well-recognised indicators of average and variability, and we stressed the importance of providing variability statistics alongside average statistics in Chapter 3. You will also see that whereas the mean ranks present your scores as a number, this number means little to the reader. However, the median presents you with a score that is meaningful within the variable as it presents a score that can be interpreted within the scores assigned to the original variable.

It means a little more work, but is worth it (though at this stage it may be useful to ask your lecturer for guidance).

So, let us do this for the previous example: examining whether there are statistically significant differences between mothers who had children who were their firstborn, and mothers for whom their child was not their firstborn, and their belief that they can protect their child from measles, mumps and rubella without the MMR jab. What we need to do is replace the mean ranks with the median and semi-interquartile range statistics. We don't have to perform the Mann–Whitney *U* test again; rather we need to work out median and variability scores, and put them in place of the mean rank scores.

To work out the median and semi-interquartile range (SIQR) in the easiest way, we need to do something a little different in SPSS for Windows. Go to SPSS for Windows (using the child branch dataset), click on **Analyze**, click on **Descriptive Statistics** and select **Explore**. Put the variable **protectMMR** (whether the person believes they can protect their child) into the **Dependent List** box, and put the **firstch** (whether the child is their first) into the **Factor list** box. Click on the **Statistics** button and click on the box next to **Percentiles** (and make sure the box next to **Descriptives** is ticked). Press **Continue** and then **OK**. You will get a printout with about four boxes, but we want you to concentrate on the two boxes shown in the figures below.

Descriptives

Is s/he your first child?				Statistic	Std. Error
I can protect my child from exposure to measles, mumps and rubella without the MMR jab	No	Mean		3.00	.459
		95% Confidence Interval for Mean	Lower Bound	2.04	
			Upper Bound	3.96	
		5% Trimmed Mean		2.72	
		Median		3.00	
		Variance		4.211	
		Std. Deviation		2.052	
		Minimum		1	
		Maximum		10	
		Range		9	
		Interquartile Range		1	
		Skewness		2.355	.512
		Kurtosis		6.860	.992
	Yes	Mean		4.05	.426
		95% Confidence Interval for Mean	Lower Bound	3.16	
			Upper Bound	4.94	
		5% Trimmed Mean		4.00	
		Median		4.00	
		Variance		3.629	
		Std. Deviation		1.905	
		Minimum		1	
		Maximum		8	
		Range		7	
		Interquartile Range		2	
		Skewness		.022	.512
		Kurtosis		-.141	.992

Median average score for women for whom the child is *not* their first child (3.00)

Median average score for women for whom the child is their first child (4.00)

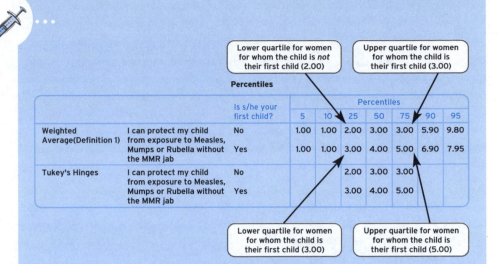

First of all is the median for each group. The median is in the **Descriptives** box, and we have highlighted the median in the figure. The median for mothers for whom the child is their first child and who believe that they can protect their child from measles, mumps and rubella without the MMR jab is 4.00. The median for mothers for whom the child is *not* their first child and who believe that they can protect their child from measles, mumps and rubella without the MMR jab is 3.00.

Second is the semi-interquartile range (an indicator of variability) for each median statistic. You need to do a bit of simple mathematics to work this out and we did this in Chapter 3. First you need to subtract the value at the lower quartile (25th percentile) from the value at the upper quartile (75th percentile) and divide this result by 2. So for our mothers for whom the child is their first child we would subtract 3 (lower quartile) from 5 (upper quartile), which would be 2, and divide this by 2. So 2 divided by 2 is 1. So the semi-interquartile range of mothers for whom the child is their first child is 1. For our mothers for whom the child is *not* their first child, we would subtract 2 (lower quartile) from 3 (upper quartile) which would be 1, and divide this by 2. So 1 divided by 2 is 0.5. So the semi-interquartile range for mothers for whom the child is *not* their first child is 0.5.

We would now rewrite our previous analysis as the following:

A Mann–Whitney *U* test was used to examine statistically significant differences between mothers who had children who were their firstborn, and mothers for whom their child was not their firstborn, and their belief that they can protect their child from measles, mumps and rubella without the MMR jab. Mothers for whom the child was their firstborn (median = 4, SIQR = 1) were found to score statistically significantly higher ($U = 121.00$, $p < 0.05$) than mothers for whom the child was not their firstborn (median = 3, SIQR = 0.5). This finding suggests that mothers with children, for whom it is their first child, believe that they can protect their child from measles, mumps and rubella without the MMR jab more so than mothers with children for whom it is not their first child.

Box 8.8 Point to consider

Calculating the Mann-Whitney *U* test by hand

In this example we're going to use a fairly straightforward example. A sample of 14 parents (7 males and 7 females) was asked to respond to the following statement: 'I think my child's having the MMR jab is important'. Responses were scored on a five-point scale: 1 = Not at all, 2 = Slightly, 3 = A little, 4 = Quite a bit, 5 = A lot. This example will determine whether there is a significant difference between men and women in their attitude to whether the MMR jab is important. We are making no specific predictions regarding whether men or women differ, and therefore it is a two-tailed prediction.

Males	Score	Overall rank	Females	Score	Overall rank
1	2	3 (Step 1)	1	4	10.5 (Step 1)
2	3	6.5 (Step 1)	2	2	3 (Step 1)
3	2	3 (Step 1)	3	4	10.5 (Step 1)
4	3	6.5 (Step 1)	4	5	13.5 (Step 1)
5	1	1 (Step 1)	5	5	13.5 (Step 1)
6	3	6.5 (Step 1)	6	4	10.5 (Step 1)
7	4	10.5 (Step 1)	7	3	6.5 (Step 1)

Step 1. Rank all the scores in order, assigning 1 to the lowest. With ranks that are equal, add the next ranks together and divide by the number of respondents who have this rank. For example, male respondents 1 and 3 have the second highest rank, and so does female respondent 2. So add ranks 2, 3, 4 and divide by the number of respondents, 3, so $2 + 3 + 4 = 9$, and $9/3 = 3$.

Step 2. Add up all the ranks for men:

$3 + 6.5 + 3 + 6.5 + 1 + 6.5 + 10.5 = 37$

Step 3. Add up all the ranks for women:

$10.5 + 3 + 10.5 + 13.5 + 13.5 + 10.5 + 6.5 = 68$

Step 4. Multiply the number of men by the number of women:

$7 \times 7 = 49$

Step 5. Multiply the number of men by (the number of men +1) and then divide this total by 2:

$7 \times (7 + 1)/2 = 7 \times 8/2 = 56/2 = 28$

Step 6. Multiply the number of women by (the number of women +1) and then divide this total by 2:

$7 \times (7 + 1)/2 = 7 \times 8/2 = 56/2 = 28$

Step 7. Add your finding for step 4 to your finding for step 5 and minus your findings for step 2:

$49 + 28 - 37 = 77 - 37 = 40$

Step 8. Add your finding for step 4 to your finding for step 6 and minus your finding for step 3:

$49 + 28 - 68 = 77 - 68 = 9$

Step 9. Select the smaller from steps 7 and 8. This is your *U* value.

Step 8 is smaller. $U = 9$

To work out whether the result is significant, find the column and row in the table below that are equal to the sample size (*N*). Our sample comprised seven males and seven females, so we read down column $N = 7$ and across row $N = 7$ to the box where they meet. This is highlighted in the table.

- The first value in each box is one-tailed test at 0.005, two-tailed test at 0.01.
- The second value in each box is one-tailed test at 0.01, two-tailed test at 0.02.
- The third value in each box is one-tailed test at 0.025, two-tailed test at 0.05.
- The fourth value in each box is one-tailed test at 0.05, two-tailed test at 0.10.

		Males (Sample 1)				
	-	4	5	6	7	8
Females	4	-, -, 0, 1	-, 0, 1, 2	0, 1, 2, 3	0, 1, 3, 4	1, 2, 4, 5
(sample 2)	5	-, 0, 1, 2	0, 1, 2, 4	1, 2, 3, 5	1, 3, 5, 6	2, 4, 6, 8
	6	0, 1, 2, 3	1, 2, 3, 5	2, 3, 5, 7	3, 4, 6, 8	4, 6, 8, 10
	7	0, 1, 3, 4	1, 3, 5, 6	3, 4, 6, 8	4, 6, 8, 11	6, 7, 10, 13
	8	1, 2, 4, 5	2, 4, 6, 8	4, 6, 8, 10	6, 7, 10, 13	7, 9, 13, 15

For our *U* statistic to be significant, *U* has to be lower than the number in the box. Our research is two-tailed and has to be significant at least at the 0.05 level. $U = 9$, and is higher than the third value, which is the 0.05 level for the two-tailed test, therefore it is not significant. If *U* had been 7, it would have been significant at the $p < 0.05$ level.

Comparing occasions: tests that compare the same subjects on a continuous variable on two occasions

The second set of tests we are going to introduce are similar to the previous two tests in that they compare differences between two sets of scores. The last set of statistical tests compared two different groups (for example, males and females) and their scores on the same variable. However, this set of tests compares the same variable on two different occasions.

Therefore this time, the tests compare the same group of people on a continuous variable of two occasions, for example self-reported pain before and after a drug trial, or changes in health before and after leaving hospital.

The two tests we are going to introduce to you here are the paired-samples *t*-test and the Wilcoxon sign-ranks test. These two tests are very similar in nature. The major difference between them is that the paired-samples *t*-test is used when the continuous variable administered on two occasions comprises parametric data, whereas the Wilcoxon sign-ranks test is used when the continuous variable administered on two occasions comprises non-parametric data.

Comparing occasions, test number 1: paired-samples *t*-test (parametric test)

The paired-samples *t*-test is used to examine the differences between scores on two continuous variables that you wish to treat as parametric data. The important difference between this test and the Pearson product–moment correlation coefficient is that, whereas the Pearson test establishes whether two different variables are correlated, the paired-samples *t*-test seeks to establish whether scores on the *same* variable, administered to the same sample on two occasions, statistically significantly differ. The paired-samples *t*-test does this by comparing the average mean scores of the same participants in two conditions, or at two points in time.

To illustrate the paired-samples *t*-test we will use the data from the mental health branch dataset that is taken from a fictitious clinical trial. In this dataset 40 schizophrenic patients are about to take the antipsychotic medication olanzapine. Researchers are interested in finding out whether a daily dosage of olanzapine will have an immediate effect on patients' psychotic symptoms. Therefore, researchers have devised a checklist that is used by doctors to assess the patients' levels in six areas: paranoia, auditory hallucinations, visual hallucinations, delusions of grandeur, disorders of streams of thought and severity of their catatonia. Each aspect of the checklist is scored on a four-point scale: 0 = Non-existent, 1 = Mild, 2 = Moderate and 3 = Severe. Responses

Box 8.9 Point to consider

Different names for the paired-samples *t*-test

The paired-samples *t*-test goes under a number of different names. Sometimes the test is referred to as the related *t*-test, related samples *t*-test, paired test, dependent groups *t*-test, *t*-test for related measures, correlated *t*-test, matched-groups *t*-test and, most importantly for our needs, the paired-samples *t*-test in SPSS for Windows. Don't worry. These are just different terms for the same test. However, one point to note is that the matched-groups *t*-test is so named because the test is sometimes used under other circumstances. Sometimes researchers cannot administer the same measure twice to the same sample, and instead have to use two samples. Here, researchers will try to match their sample in as many ways as possible (it may be by variables such as sex, age, educational attainment, length in treatment, and so forth) to simulate using the same sample. On these occasions you will find researchers using a related *t*-test, referring to it as a matched-groups sample.

are then totalled to provide an overall checklist score, with higher scores indicating a greater level of psychotic symptoms (with possible scores ranging from 0 to 18). Researchers want to test whether the dosages of olanzapine will decrease patients' psychotic symptoms scores (and please forgive the lack of a control group, for now we are only looking at the data for the people who were administered the drug). Therefore, they administered all 40 patients the psychotic symptoms checklist before the dosage, and then after the trial had finished they administered the checklist to all the patients again. We will now use SPSS Windows to see whether olanzapine had a statistically significant effect on reducing the patients' psychotic symptoms.

Performing the paired-samples t-test on SPSS for Windows

Load up the mental health branch dataset and select the paired-samples *t*-test by clicking on the **Analyze** pull-down menu, then **Compare Means** and then **Paired-Samples T test…** . Then, and be careful here, highlight the two variable names **Checklist1** and **Checklist2** in the left-hand box (by clicking on them with the mouse). You will see that both of the variables appear in the **Current Selection** box, next to **Variable 1:** and **Variable 2:** in the bottom left-hand corner (Figure 8.8). Then, and only then, click on the arrow button to transfer the two variables into the **Paired Variables** box.

Click on **OK** to run the *t*-test. The output should look like Figure 8.9.

In this output, we have all the information we need to interpret whether a statistically significant difference occurs between scores for the two administrations of the checklist scale. Again, remember to *describe* and then *decide*.

Using 'describe and decide' to interpret the paired-samples t-test

From the output in Figure 8.9, you will need to consider three things:

- *Mean scores and standard deviations*. These are the basis of our description. We note both the mean scores (with the standard deviation) and which mean score for which administration is higher.
- *The t value*. The test statistic.
- *The Sig. (2-tailed)*. The significance level. This is the probability level given to the current findings. The significance level tells the researcher whether the difference between the means is significant. Remember, if this figure is below the $p = 0.05$ or $p = 0.01$ criterion, then the finding is statistically significant. If this figure is above 0.05, then the findings are not statistically significant.

We can see from Figure 8.9 that the mean score on the first administration of the psychotic symptoms checklist before the use of olanzapine is 8.73 (with a standard deviation of 3.23) and the average mean score on the psychotic symptoms checklist after the use of olanzapine on the second administration is 7.58 (with a standard deviation

(a)

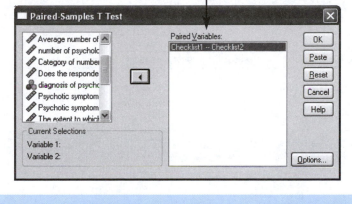

You need to click on the two variables first and they will show up in the **Current Selections** box. Then you need to transfer them both across to the **Paired Variables:** box with the arrow button

(b)

Figure 8.8 Paired-Samples T Test window

of 2.7) (note that all these figures are rounded to two decimal places). We note here that the psychotic symptoms checklist scores for the second administration are lower than for the first administration. The t value for the statistic is 3.851. This tells us very little at this stage. However, the significance level is $p = 0.000$. This is smaller than 0.01. Therefore, we conclude that a statistically significant difference for mean scores exists between the two administrations of the psychotic symptoms checklist. This suggests that the dosage of olanzapine had a statistically significant effect on lowering psychotic symptoms among the present sample.

Using 'describe and decide' to report the paired-samples t-test

The next stage is to report these statistics. There is a formal way of reporting the paired-samples t-test, which comprises two elements. First there is a formal statement of your statistics, which must include the following:

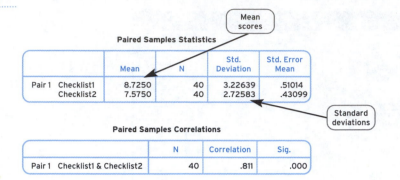

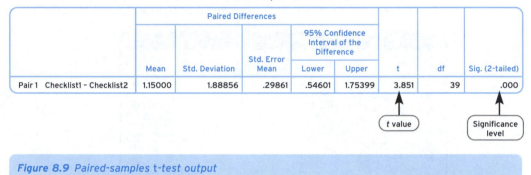

Figure 8.9 *Paired-samples t-test output*

- *The test statistic.* Each test has a symbol for its statistic. The paired-samples *t*-test has the symbol *t*. Therefore, in your write-up you must include what *t* is equal to. In the example, $t = 3.85$.

- *The degrees of freedom.* This concept was introduced in Chapter 6, and is tradition-ally reported (though it is worth noting that it is not always reported). For the paired-samples *t*-test, the degrees of freedom equal the size of your sample -1. Here, the minus 1 represents minus 1 for the sample, because you have asked only one set of respondents. This figure is placed between the *t* and the equals sign and is written in brackets. Here, the degrees of freedom are 39 (size of sample $= 40$, minus $1 = 39$). Therefore, $t(39) = 3.85$.

- *The probability.* Remember there are two ways to report the probability:

  - The traditional way is in relation to whether your probability value is below 0.05 or 0.01 (statistically significant) or above 0.05 (not statistically significant). Here, you use less than (<) or greater than (>) the criteria levels. You state these criteria by reporting whether $p < 0.05$ (statistically significant), $p < 0.01$ (statistically significant) or $p > 0.05$ (not statistically significant). In the example above, as

$p = 0.000$, we would write $p < 0.01$ and place this after the reporting of the *t* value. Therefore, with our findings, $t(39) = 3.85$, $p < 0.01$.

- Statisticians and researchers have started reporting the *p* value as it is; in our case $p = 0.000$. However, it must be appreciated that the probability value that is reported as '.000' in SPSS appears as such because SPSS typically reports only to three decimal places, so actually '.000' means a value less than 0.0005. Consequently you would do better to report *p* as $p < 0.0005$. Therefore, we would write $t(39) = 3.85$, $p < 0.0005$.

This must then be incorporated into the report to help the reader understand and conceptualise your findings. In writing up the report use the 'describe and decide' rule to inform the reader of your finding:

- Remind the reader of the two variables you are examining.
- Say which mean score is the higher.
- Tell the reader whether the finding is statistically significant or not.

You can use all the information above to write a fairly simple sentence which conveys your findings succinctly but effectively. Therefore, using the findings above we might report:

Psychotic symptoms checklist after the use of olanzapine

A paired-samples *t*-test was used to examine whether olanzapine had a statistically significant effect on psychotic symptoms. A statistically significant difference ($t(39) = 3.85$, $p < 0.0005$) was found for mean scores on a psychotic symptoms checklist, with mean scores for psychotic symptoms being statistically significantly lower for the second administration of the psychotic symptoms checklist

Box 8.10 Point to consider

Writing up a non-significant result for paired-samples *t*-test: an example

A paired-samples *t*-test was used to examine whether olanzapine had a significant effect on psychotic symptoms. No significant differences ($t(39) = 1.30$, $p = 0.66$ [or $p > 0.05$]) were found for scores on a checklist of psychotic symptoms (mean = 7.34, S.D. = 1.8) before the administration of olanzapine, and scores on the same checklist of psychotic symptoms after the administration of olanzapine (mean = 7.26, S.D. = 1.9). The present findings suggest that olanzapine does not have a significant effect on psychotic symptoms.

(mean = 7.58, S.D. = 2.7) than for the first administration of the psychotic symptoms checklist (mean = 8.73, S.D. = 3.2). The current findings suggest that olanzapine reduces psychotic symptoms.

Again, you will come across different ways of writing up tests, but you will find all the information included above in any write-up. If you want to expand your knowledge a little, read Boxes 8.10 and 8.11.

Box 8.11 Point to consider

Calculating the paired-samples *t*-test by hand

Five students are due to sit a pre-entrance nursing exam. The researcher is interested in finding out whether anxiety levels change before and after the exam. The same scale is administered to the students before and after the exam. The scale asks students to rate their current anxiety level on a scale of 1 (not anxious at all) to 10 (very anxious). The following scores were obtained.

Student	Anxiety level before the exam	Anxiety level after the exam
1	7	4
2	5	6
3	6	4
4	7	3
5	8	3

Step 1. Find the mean score for the variable 'Anxiety level before the exam':

$$\frac{7 + 5 + 6 + 7 + 8}{5} = \frac{33}{5} = 6.6$$

Step 2. Find the mean score for the variable 'Anxiety level after the exam':

$$\frac{4 + 6 + 4 + 3 + 3}{5} = \frac{20}{5} = 4.0$$

Step 3. Subtract the smaller value from steps 1 and 2 from the other:

$$6.6 - 4.0 = 2.6$$

Step 4. Subtract each number in the column 'Anxiety level after the exam' from its partner number in the column 'Anxiety level before the exam':

$$7 - 4 = 3, \quad 5 - 6 = -1, \quad 6 - 4 = 2, \quad 7 - 3 = 4, \quad 8 - 3 = 5$$

Step 5. Square each number calculated in step 4, and then add them together.

$3 \times 3 = 9$, $-1 \times -1 = 1$, $2 \times 2 = 4$, $4 \times 4 = 16$, $5 \times 5 = 25 \Rightarrow 9 + 1 + 4 + 16 + 25 = 55$

Step 6. Add up all the numbers calculated in step 4 (take minus signs into account):

$3 + -1 + 2 + 4 + 5 = 13$

Anxiety level before the exam	Anxiety level after the exam	Step 4	Step 5	Step 6
7	4	3	9	3
5	6	−1	1	−1
6	4	2	4	2
7	3	4	16	4
8	3	5	25	5
			55	13

Step 7. Square the value found in step 6:

$13 \times 13 - 169$

Step 8. Count the number of pairs of scores = 5.

Step 9. Subtract 1 from the number of pairs of scores (this also gives the degrees of freedom):

$5 - 1 = 4$

Step 10. Multiply the values found in steps 8 and 9:

$5 \times 4 = 20$

Step 11. Divide the number found in step 7 by the number found in step 10:

$169/20 = 8.45$

Step 12. Subtract the value found in step 11 from that found in step 5 and divide this number by the number found in step 10:

$(55 - 8.45)/20 = 2.33$

Step 13. Square root the value obtained in step 12:

$\sqrt{2.33} = 1.53$

Step 14. Divide the value found in step 3 by the value found in step 13. This is your *t* value:

$t = 2.6/1.53 = 1.699$

Use the table below to determine the significance of your result.

	Significance levels for two-tailed test				
	0.05	0.025	0.01	0.0005	0.00005
	Significance levels for one-tailed test				
d.f.	0.10	0.05	0.02	0.01	0.001
1	6.314	12.71	31.82	63.66	636.6
2	2.92	4.303	6.969	9.925	31.6
3	2.353	3.182	4.541	5.841	12.92
4	2.132	2.776	3.747	4.604	8.610
5	2.015	2.571	3.365	4.032	6.869

The degrees of freedom were calculated in step 9 and equal 4.

We will use a two-tailed test because the researcher has not predicted that anxiety changes in any particularly direction. We will also use a significance level of 0.05. With degrees of freedom = 4, and using a two-tailed test, at a significance level of 0.05 the value to be compared is 2.132. Our *t* is 1.699. This is smaller than 2.132 and therefore we would conclude that there is no statistically significant difference in anxiety levels for students before and after the exam.

Comparing occasions, test number 2: Wilcoxon sign-ranks test (non-parametric test)

The Wilcoxon sign-ranks test is the non-parametric alternative to the paired-samples *t*-test. It is used when you have measured the same continuous variable on two occasions among the same respondents and you do not wish to treat your continuous data as parametric.

Whereas the paired-samples *t*-test was based on examining whether statistically significant differences occur between mean scores (with standard deviations), the Wilcoxon sign-ranks test, because the data are ranked, is based on examining statistically significant differences between average ranks.

Performing the Wilcoxon sign-ranks test in SPSS for Windows

You probably have a grasp of these comparison tests by now. Nevertheless, to illustrate the Wilcoxon sign-ranks test, let us use a fairly simple example.

Open the adult dataset. You will remember this dataset relates to a sample of 74 elderly people and issues to do with their health and their mobility after a fall. Within this dataset are two variables that relate to respondents' views of the usefulness of walking frames provided to them by the NHS. All 74 respondents were asked to rate the usefulness of their walking frames on a ten-point scale ranging from 1 (very dissatisfied) to 10 (very satisfied).

The local health authority then funded a scheme by which all walking frames were replaced with new ones. To see how successful the scheme was, all respondents were asked the same question again. We will now use SPSS for Windows to assess how successful the scheme was.

There are two variables that correspond to this study: **walkingframes1**, the first time the measure was administered and **walkingframes2**, the second time the measure was administered.

The first thing we could do is to show you that we should be using a non-parametric test. Figure 8.10 shows the histograms for both variables. As you can see, one of these variables, **walkingframes2**, shows a negative skew, with responses weighted to the higher scoring responses. To examine this further we could look at the skewness statistics. For the first administration of the walking frame question, the skewness statistic is −0.642. For the second administration, it is −1.107. Therefore, although with the first administration of the question the skewness is below the criterion of +1 or −1, the second administration shows the skewness statistic is above the criterion, and if one of the variables is skewed then this is a reason to perform a non-parametric test.

To perform the Wilcoxon sign-ranks test in SPSS for Windows, go to the **Analyze** pull-down menu and click on **Nonparametric Tests**. Next click on **2 Related Samples**. Highlight the two variable names in the left-hand box, and they will appear in the **Current Selections** box below. Then move them into the **Test Pair(s) List:** box by clicking on the arrow button (see Figure 8.11). Make sure the **Wilcoxon** box is ticked and then click on **OK**. You will then get an output like that in Figure 8.12.

In this output we have all the information we need to interpret whether a statistically significant difference occurs between scores for the two administrations of the walking frame variables. Again, remember to *describe* and then *decide*.

Using 'describe and decide' to interpret the Wilcoxon sign-ranks test

From the output in Figure 8.12, you will need to consider three things:

● *Mean ranks*. These are the basis of our description. Here, lower ranks mean lower scores (remember 2, 5, 7, 10, 13 would be ranked 1, 2, 3, 4, 5). We note both the mean

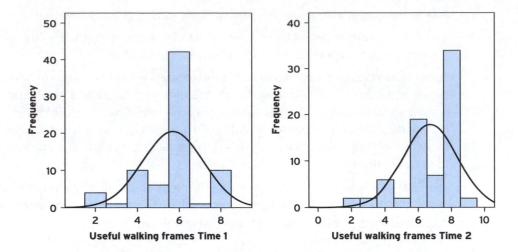

Figure 8.10 *Histograms and skewness statistics showing distributions for the question relating to usefulness of walking frames on two occasions*

ranks and then which mean rank is higher. In the Wilcoxon sign-ranks test output in SPSS for Windows this is expressed in a certain way. If you look at the table you will see that in the N column of the ranks table there are three letters, a, b and c. These correspond to some statements under the table:

● *The first is a.* This refers to the number of ranks in the sample in which Useful walking frames Time 1 is greater than Useful walking frames Time 2 (although it is referred to in the table as Time 2 < [less than] Time 1).

● *The second is b.* This refers to the number of ranks in the sample in which Useful walking frames Time 2 is greater than Useful walking frames Time 1.

● *The third is c.* This refers to the number of times that the ranks for Useful walking frames Time 1 and Time 2 are the same.

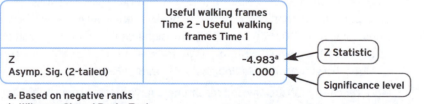

Figure 8.11 *Two-Related-Samples Tests window*

Ranks

		N	Mean Rank	Sum of Ranks
Useful walking frames Time 2 – Useful walking frames Time 1	Negative Ranks	9[a]	26.50	238.50
	Positive Ranks	49[b]	30.05	1472.50
	Ties	16[c]		
	Total	74		

a. Useful walking frames Time 2 < Useful walking frames Time 1
b. Useful walking frames Time 2 > Useful walking frames Time 1
c. Useful walking frames Time 2 = Useful walking frames Time 1

Number of ranks

Mean rank

Test Statistics[b]

	Useful walking frames Time 2 – Useful walking frames Time 1
Z	-4.983[a]
Asymp. Sig. (2-tailed)	.000

Z Statistic

Significance level

a. Based on negative ranks
b. Wilcoxon Signed Ranks Test

Figure 8.12 *Output for the Wilcoxon sign-ranks statistic comparing attitudes towards the usefulness of walking frames before and after a local health authority initiative*

For our analysis we are interested in a and b, and in obtaining an average score for each occasion the question was asked. For time 1 we use the mean ranks in line a, negative ranks. For time 2 we use the mean ranks in line b, positive ranks. So, the mean rank for Useful walking frames Time 1 is 26.50. The mean rank for the Useful walking frames Time 2 is 30.05. Here, we note that average ranks for the second administration are higher than those for the first administration.

We then need to determine whether these average (mean) ranks are statistically significantly different. Therefore we need the next two statistics.

- *The z value*. The test statistic.
- *The Asymp Sig. (2-tailed)*. The significance level. This is the probability level given to the current findings. The significance level indicates whether there are statistically significant differences between the mean scores. Remember, if this figure is below the $p = 0.05$ or $p = 0.01$ criterion, then the finding is statistically significant. If this figure is above 0.05, then the findings are not statistically significant.

The *z* value for the statistic is -4.983. This tells us very little at this stage. However, the significance level is $p = 0.000$. This is smaller than 0.01 and so we conclude that there is a statistically significant difference for mean ranks between the two administrations of the questions about the usefulness of the walking frames provided.

Using 'describe and decide' to report the Wilcoxon sign-ranks test

The next stage is to report these statistics. There is a formal way of reporting the Wilcoxon sign-ranks test, which comprises two elements. First there is a formal statement of your statistics, which must include the following:

- *The test statistic*. Each test has a symbol for its statistic. The Wilcoxon sign-ranks test has the symbol *z*. Therefore, in your write-up you must include what *z* is equal to. In the example $z = -4.98$ (to two decimal places).
- *The probability*. As usual, this can be reported in one of two ways:
  - The traditional way is to report whether your probability value is below 0.05 or 0.01 (statistically significant) or above 0.05 (not statistically significant). Here, you use less than (<) or greater than (>) the criteria levels. You state these criteria by reporting whether $p < 0.05$ (statistically significant), $p < 0.01$ (statistically significant) or $p > 0.05$ (not statistically significant). So, in the example above, as $p = 0.000$, we would write $p < 0.01$ and place this after the reporting of the *z* value. Therefore, with our findings, $z = -4.98$, $p < 0.01$.
  - More recently, statisticians and researchers have started reporting the *p* value as it is; in our case $p = 0.000$. Therefore, we would write, $z = -4.98$, $p = 0.000$.

This must then be incorporated into the text, to help the reader understand and conceptualise your findings. In writing up the text, use the 'describe and decide' rule to inform the reader of your finding:

- Remind the reader of the two variables you are examining.
- Say which mean score is the higher.
- Tell the reader whether the finding is statistically significant or not.

You can use all the information above to write a fairly simple sentence which conveys your findings succinctly but effectively. Therefore, using the findings above we might report:

> A Wilcoxon sign-ranks test was used to examine statistically significant differences between views of usefulness of walking frames before and after a local health authority initiative to update all walking frames. The view of the usefulness of walking frames was statistically significantly higher ($z = -4.98$; $p = 0.000$) after the local health authority initiative (mean rank = 30.05) than before the local health authority initiative (mean rank = 26.50). The findings suggest that the introduction of new walking frames met with a favourable response by respondents.

Box 8.12 Point to consider

Writing up a non-significant result for a Wilcoxon sign-ranks test: an example

A Wilcoxon sign-ranks test was used to examine significant differences between views of usefulness of walking frames before and after a local health authority initiative to update all walking frames. There was no significant difference ($z = 2.76$; $p = 0.76$ [or $p > 0.05$]) between views after the local health authority had introduced a new set of walking frames (mean rank = 9.32) and views before the local health authority initiative (mean rank = 9.56). The findings suggest that the introduction of new walking frames had no effect on the perception of the usefulness of walking frames.

Again, you will come across different ways of writing tests, but you will find all the information included above in any write-up. However, if you want to expand your knowledge a little then read Boxes 8.12–8.14.

Effect sizes

You may remember that in Chapter 7 we talked about effect sizes with correlations. Effect sizes can be used to estimate the magnitude or the importance, rather than just relying on significance. You will remember that an effect size of 0.2 was considered small, 0.5 medium and 0.8 large.

Box 8.13 Point to consider

Medians rather than mean ranks for the Wilcoxon sign-ranks test

It doesn't quite end here with the Wilcoxon sign-ranks test. Like the Mann-Whitney *U* test before, we suggest using the median and the semi-interquartile range (see Box 8.7 for a fuller explanation).

Let us do this for the last example, examining statistically significant differences between views of usefulness of walking frames before and after a local health authority initiative to update all walking frames. What we need to do is replace the mean ranks with the median and semi-interquartile range statistics.

To work out the median and semi-interquartile range (SIQR) you need to return to the adult dataset, click on **Analyze**, select **Descriptive Statistics** and then **Frequencies**. You need to transfer the two walking frame variables (**walkingframes1** and **walkingframes2**) into the **Variable(s):** box. You then need to click on **Statistics** and click on the boxes next to **median** and **quartiles**. Hit **Continue** and then **OK**. You will get a printout, but we want you to focus on the following statistics:

		Useful walking frames Time 1	Useful walking frames Time 2
N	Valid	74	74
	Missing	0	0
Median		6.00	7.00
Percentiles	25	4.00	6.00
	50	6.00	7.00
	75	6.00	8.00

First is the median for each occasion. The median for the view of the usefulness of walking frames *before* the initiative was 6.00. The median for the view of the usefulness of walking frames after the initiative was 7.00.

Second is the semi-interquartile range (an indicator of variability) for each median statistic. You need to do a bit of simple mathematics to work this out and we did this in Chapter 3 (and in Box 8.7). To work out the semi-interquartile range you need to subtract the value at the lower quartile (25th percentile) from the value at the upper quartile (75th percentile) and divide this result by 2. So, for the view of the usefulness of walking frames *before* the initiative we would subtract 4 (lower quartile) from 6 (upper quartile), which would be 2, and divide this by 2.

...

So 2 divided by 2 is 1, so the semi-interquartile range for the view of the usefulness of walking frames *before* the initiative is 1 (SIQR = 1).

For our view of the usefulness of walking frames *after* the initiative we would subtract 6 (lower quartile) from 8 (upper quartile), which would be 2 and divide this by 2. So 2 divided by 2 is 1, so the semi-interquartile range view of the usefulness of walking frames *after* the initiative is 1.

Therefore we would rewrite our previous analysis as follows:

> A Wilcoxon sign-ranks test was used to examine statistically significant differences between views of usefulness of walking frames before and after a local health authority initiative to update all walking frames. The view of the usefulness of walking frames was statistically significantly higher ($z = -4.98$, $p < 0.01$) after the local health authority initiative (median = 7, SIQR = 1) than before the local health authority initiative (median = 6, SIQR = 1). The findings suggest that the introduction of new walking frames met with a favourable response by respondents.

Box 8.14 Point to consider

Calculating the Wilcoxon sign-ranks test by hand

The local health authority are monitoring how well seven of its residents are in one of its local nursing homes. The sample of seven residents was asked to complete the same measure twice on two occasions, six months apart. The measure 'How often do you feel ill?' was scored 1 = Not at all, 2 = Very rarely, 3 = Sometimes, 4 = Monthly, 5 = Weekly, 6 = Daily, 7 = More than once every day.

Respondent	Illness time 1	Illness time 2	Difference	Rank order of differences
1	1	2	−1 (Step 1)	1 (Step 2)
2	4	2	+2 (Step 1)	2.5 (Step 2)
3	4	1	+3 (Step 1)	4 (Step 2)
4	5	5	0 (Step 1)	
5	7	3	+4 (Step 1)	5 (Step 2)
6	2	4	−2 (Step 1)	2.5 (Step 2)
7	1	7	−6 (Step 1)	6 (Step 2)

Step 1. Work out the differences between each pair of scores.

$1 - 2 = -1$, $4 - 2 = 2$, $4 - 1 = +3$, $5 - 5 = 0$, $7 - 3 = 4$, $2 - 4 = -2$, $1 - 7 = -6$

Step 2. Rank the order of differences from lowest value to highest values, ignoring 0 (as with respondent 4) and ignoring + and − signs. With ranks that are equal, add the next ranks together and divide by the number of respondents who have this rank. For example, respondents 2 and 6 have the second highest rank so add 2 (the next rank) + 3 (the next rank after that) and divide by the number of respondents: $(2 + 3)/2 = 5/2 = 2.5$, so each person gets a rank of 2.5.

Step 3. Add the ranks of the + values and − values:

+ values: $2.5 + 4 + 5 = 11.5$ − values: $1 + 2.5 + 6 = 9.5$

Step 4. The smaller set of scores is your Wilcoxon sign-ranks value (z). Here $z = 9.5$

To work out whether the result is significant, we use the table below. As, we have made no prediction about direction of the differences between the scores on both the variables, we use the two-tailed test. Find the row that is equal to the sample size, 7, and then find the number in this row that z is bigger than. If z is bigger than all the numbers, then z is not significant.

	Significance levels for one-tailed test			
	0.05	0.025	0.01	0.0001
	Significance levels for two-tailed test			
Sample size	0.10	0.05	0.02	0.0002
5	$z < 0$			
6	2	0		
7	3	2	0	
8	5	3	2	1
9	8	5	3	3

One handy thing you may want to know is that effect size can be calculated for tests of difference. What you may not want to know is that you have to calculate it largely by hand with the help of SPSS for Windows, as unfortunately SPSS for Windows doesn't supply this statistic for you.

To calculate the effect size for differences between two sets of scores, subtract the mean of one set of scores from the mean of the other set of scores, and then divide it by the standard deviation statistic for the total scores. This will give you your effect size.

Let us calculate the effect size for some variables in the adult branch dataset. In this dataset we have a record of the number of falls someone has had (**Numberfalls**), and we have also recorded whether they have problems with their vision (**visimpair**). Therefore, we could be interested in finding out whether visual impairment is a factor in falling. Therefore, we would do an independent-samples *t*-test to compare those people who haven't got a visual impairment (group 1) with those who have got a visual impairment (group 2) on the number of falls they have (see Figure 8.13). Do be aware that you don't have to do an independent-samples *t*-test; all you need is the mean for the two sets of scores.

As you would no doubt confirm, it is clear from this that visually impaired people have statistically significantly more falls than people who are not visually impaired. However, what we also need to do is find the effect size. We have nearly all the information here to do that; there is just one piece missing: the overall standard deviation for the **Numberfalls** variable (we only have the group standard deviations here). This we can get from the descriptive statistics procedure (Figure 8.14).

Group Statistics

	Has the person got visual impairment?	N	Mean	Std. Deviation	Std. Error Mean
Numberfalls	No	32	2.1563	.91966	.16257
	Yes	42	2.9762	1.35229	.20866

Independent Samples Test

		Levene's Test for Equality of Variances		t-test for Equality of Means						95% Confidence Interval of the Difference	
		F	Sig.	t	df	Sig. (2-tailed)	Mean Difference	Std. Error Difference		Lower	Upper
Numberfalls	Equal variances assumed	6.497	.013	-2.947	72	.004	-.81994	.27818		-1.37449	-.26539
	Equal variances not assumed			-3.100	71.190	.003	-.81994	.26452		-1.34735	-.29253

Figure 8.13 *Independent-samples t-test comparing visually impaired groups on the number of falls they have suffered*

Descriptive Statistics

	N	Minimum	Maximum	Mean	Std. Deviation
Numberfalls	74	1.00	5.00	2.6216	1.24639
Valid N (listwise)	74				

Figure 8.14 Standard deviation information for the **Numberfalls** variable

Now we have all the information we need. So, we first subtract the mean of one group from the mean of the other (it doesn't matter which way round), but let us take the smallest from the largest, so $2.9762 - 2.1563 = 0.8199$. And then we divide that number by the overall standard deviation, 1.24639.

So 0.8199 divided by $1.24639 = 0.66$ (rounded up to the nearest two decimal places). This means we have an effect size of 0.66, which is medium to large. When reporting it, you call it *d*. So here $d = 0.66$.

Easy. You can also do this with the paired-samples *t*-test (although you may have to do some rearranging of data as they wouldn't all be in the same column). Nonetheless, you now know that if you do a series of *t*-tests, you can calculate the effect size to determine which is the most important finding.

Summary

In this chapter you have learnt how to perform, analyse and report four statistical tests:

✔ **Independent-samples *t*-test – this is used when you have one categorical variable with two levels, and one continuous variable that you have decided can be used in a parametric test.**

✔ **Paired-samples *t*-test – this is used when you have the same continuous variable, administered on two occasions, and you have decided the data are suitable for use in a parametric test.**

✔ **Wilcoxon sign-ranks test – this is used with a continuous variable that has been administered on two occasions, but you have decided to use the variables in a non-parametric test.**

✔ **Mann–Whitney *U* test – this is used with one categorical variable with two levels, and one continuous variable that you have decided to use in a non-parametric test.**

In this and the previous two chapters we have introduced you to a series of tests that use statistical significance. In the next chapter we are going to expand on some of the ideas that have been presented in this book by introducing some concepts that will enable you to go into greater detail when reporting your statistics and will enhance your reading of the nursing literature that contains statistics.

Self-assessment exercise

Now test your knowledge in these areas by selecting the question that is appropriate to your branch of nursing. It is worth noting that, for different datasets, some exercises are based on independent comparisons and some on dependent comparisons. Therefore, if you want to expand your self-assessment you might want to try another couple of questions from the other datasets.

Adult branch

As Graham A. Jackson (2002) notes, there are four common types of dementia: vascular, frontotemporal, Huntington's disease and normal pressure hydrocephalus. He also notes that there are many consequences of dementia, including various physical and cognitive losses encompassing decision-making abilities, self-care skills, memory and dignity.

In this dataset we have two variables that will allow us to explore this issue. The first is whether the people in our sample have been diagnosed with dementia or not (**dementia**) and the nurse's assessment of how well the person is able to make independent decisions (**abilitytomakedecisions**). Examine whether there is a statistically significant difference between patients having dementia and their ability to make decisions.

Remember to consider whether you are using an independent- or dependent-type statistical test, and whether the test uses parametric or non-parametric data. Also remember to consider average scores, and which average scores are higher.

Mental health branch

Tony Bush (2005) writes about case management in community psychiatric care, a process of psychiatric care provision that uses a structured and focused approach to assess individual patients' needs. Bush reviews the current status of case management in NHS community mental health care.

In our dataset we have two variables. The first measures the attitude of a local NHS community mental health case management team and how well the team feels they are meeting a particular patient's mental health needs (**AdequateProvision1**). The second variable also measures how well the team feels they are meeting this patient's mental health needs (**AdequateProvision2**), but six months after they had undergone a major review of the structure and administration of their case management and psychiatric care provision.

Examine whether there is a statistically significant difference between how well the team feels they are meeting the patient's needs for these two occasions.

Remember to consider whether you are using an independent- or dependent-type statistical test, and whether the test uses parametric or non-parametric data. Also remember to consider average scores, and which average scores are higher.

Learning disability branch

Roberta Astor (2001) discusses the problems of detecting pain in people with profound learning disabilities. Astor suggests that although people with profound learning difficulties show discomfort when feeling pain, they often do not understand what is happening, are unable to ask for help and information, and cannot communicate their pain verbally. Astor developed a pain assessment test for people with profound learning disabilities.

In our dataset we have some information that we can use to look at this area. The first variable is whether the person is considered to have a profound learning disability (**profound**). The second variable are scores on a pain assessment test which indicate how well the individual can understand, ask for help and communicate regarding pain (**painassessmenttest**).

Examine whether there is a statistically significant difference between those considered to have profound learning difficulties and those considered not to have profound learning difficulties and their ability to understand, ask for help and communicate regarding pain.

Remember to consider whether you are using an independent- or dependent-type statistical test, and whether the test uses parametric or non-parametric data. Also remember to consider average scores, and which average scores are higher.

Child branch

As Jane Hanley (2006) describes, post-natal depression is a common depressive illness with a variety of potential causes. She suggests that nurses need to look for the signs and symptoms of post-natal depression so that mothers with the condition are appropriately assessed and treated.

Hanley recommends the use of the Edinburgh Postnatal Depression Scale (EPDS; Cox *et al.*, 1987) designed to assess depression at six to eight weeks and at six to eight months post-natally.

We are going to look at depression levels among our sample of mothers. We have a first assessment of depression from scores on the EPDS at six to eight weeks (**EPDS1**) and a second assessment of depression from scores on the EPDS at six to eight months (**EPDS2**).

Examine whether there is a statistically significant difference between levels of post-natal depression in our sample for these two occasions.

Remember to consider whether you are using an independent- or dependent-type statistical test, and whether the test uses parametric or non-parametric data. Also remember to consider average scores, and which average scores are higher.

Further reading

We would encourage you to read the articles mentioned in the self-assessment exercise to develop ideas around these topics. They are all available free online (after registering) at the *Nursing Times* website: www.nursingtimes.net/. The references for the articles are:

Astor, R. (2001) 'Detecting pain in people with profound learning disabilities', *Nursing Times*, 97(40): 38.

Bush, T. (2005) 'Reviewing case management in community psychiatric care', *Nursing Times*, 101(38): 40–43.

Hanley, J. (2006) 'The assessment and treatment of postnatal depression', *Nursing Times*, 102(1): 24–26.

Jackson, G.A. (2002) 'Behaviour problems and assessment in dementia', *Nursing Times*, 98(47): 32.

You will be able to access the articles by typing the first author's surname or the title of the paper in the Search box on the website.

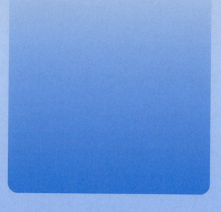

Chapter 9

Critical appraisal of analysis and reporting of inferential statistics

Key themes

✔ Critical appraisal
✔ Inferential statistics

Learning outcomes

By the end of this chapter you will be able to:

✔ Use critical appraisal to evaluate the reporting of inferential statistics

✔ Apply a critical appraisal framework to evaluate research and research articles

Introduction

Imagine . . . That you are a gerontological nurse working on a care of the older person ward. As part of your nursing team's journal club, your nursing sister has given you a task to find journal articles relating to nutrition as a risk factor for falls among older patients in the ward environment. The sister has told you that she expects you not just to look at the article's abstract but to make an informed decision about the statistics and whether or not there is a significant relationship between poor nutrition among older patients and risk of falling. You have been given an important job as it looks as if the sister will be using your findings to inform her decision whether the nutritional status of older patients should be assessed upon admission to the ward and during the patients' stays on the ward. As preparation for the journal club meeting you need to be able to do a critical appraisal of the studies into nutrition and falls among older patients. You would need to ask such questions as 'Are the authors clear about there being a relationship between these two variables?', 'How strong is the relationship? and 'Is it a statistically significant relationship?' This time you will need to use your critical appraisal skills to evaluate how inferential statistics are reported. We will be revisiting this case study scenario later in the chapter.

In recent chapters we have looked at how to carry out inferential statistics to analyse the relationships or differences between variables. In this chapter, you will be reintroduced to what critical appraisal is and how it can be used when assessing the quality of a research study. By using a critical appraisal framework, you will be in a strong position to know whether the study has been designed well and whether the inferential statistics have been correctly reported and interpreted. Through the use of case examples, we will show the usefulness of a critical appraisal framework when critiquing the statistics that have been reported in order to make inferences about data collected from a sample of participants. At the end of this chapter, you should have the skills to use the critical appraisal framework with a range of studies.

Critical appraisal revisited

Critical appraisal is a process of looking at a study in a rigorous and methodical manner. Critical appraisal is about a way of testing knowledge through looking at a study in a variety of ways. The process entails a questioning element, whereby you would systematically go through a series of questions to learn more about the strengths and limitations of a study. It also involves making an evaluation as to whether what the researchers have done is appropriate according to statistical criteria of best practice. The critical appraisal that you will be doing in this chapter follows a framework of questions intended to tap into how valid and reliable the reporting of inferential statistics has been in a study.

A critical appraisal framework for evaluating inferential statistics

The critical appraisal framework is organised into five main sections. Depending on which parts of a research report you are looking at, you will be using mainly one or other of the framework's sections. This framework covers a critical appraisal of an entire report, which would normally be organised into the four main sections of Introduction, Method, Results and Discussion (although the abstract is undoubtedly an important section, this part of the report covers mainly the four major sections, but in abbreviated form). We now give an overview of the sections of the critical appraisal framework and will use excerpts from published studies to illustrate the kinds of things you need to be searching for. After we have demonstrated the principles of criticality needed in applying the framework, we present a case study of a typical research report that you might encounter when reading the nursing research literature. You will be shown a fictitious article based on analysis of the adult branch dataset available with this book. It will be your job to critically appraise this article by using the framework.

The critical appraisal framework (see Table 9.1) has been designed so that it is sufficiently general to be applied when evaluating any type of nursing research or other kinds of healthcare/health services research.

Table 9.1 The critical appraisal framework

Section 1: Hypotheses and statistical significance
Section 2: Design
Section 3: Analysis
Section 4: Reporting findings
Section 5: Interpretation and contextualisation of findings
      General observations

We will look at the finer details of each of the sections in turn and show why these elements are essential to doing a good job when critiquing a study.

Section 1: Hypotheses and statistical significance

In this section we are trying to get a clearer idea about how scientific the study can be by looking at whether the researchers generated predictions about what they would find prior to collecting the data. If the study was mainly an exploratory one without any clearly defined **hypotheses** (that is, predictions on what would be found), then it is possible that the researchers have introduced an element of bias by not basing predictions on previous research or instances of clinical practice. The authors of the research paper need to show how the hypothesis or the aims/objectives of the study arose from previous research. This is to show that the research is often based on nursing-related theory and experiences from clinical practice.

Table 9.2 Section 1 of the critical appraisal framework

Section	Where to look in the research report	What questions to ask
1. Setting the scene: hypotheses and statistical significance	Introduction and Method	● Are there explicit stated hypotheses before conducting the study?
		● Are hypotheses based on prior research or clinical practice?
		● Is there a clearly stated level of significance for interpreting significant/non-significant results?

For research to have better scientific quality it is helpful to have an explicit statement of the predicted relationship between the variables, or the difference between them, in the form of a hypothesis. Likewise, it is useful to know what the researchers have set an acceptable level of statistical significance to gauge whether such relationships or differences can be put down to chance or to a real statistical effect. Are researchers setting their significance level[1] for getting a chance result at 0.05 or 0.01? Sometimes journals insist that authors set a standard significance level and stick to it rather than change the acceptable level of significance depending on what has been obtained with the data. Such insistence is generally good practice as it prompts researchers to set these levels beforehand. Irrespective of whether the levels are set before or after the analyses have been done, you will need to check that the size of a significant or non-significant finding is reported every time an inferential statistic is mentioned. Table 9.2 highlights the main issues to focus on when addressing section 1 of the critical appraisal framework.

● Section 2: Design

Critical appraisal of how the research has been designed will involve looking out for what is said in the Method section of the report, although you may need also to scan through the Discussion section to see whether the authors have recognised any limitations of the design. For instance, it might be that the authors have carried out a cross-sectional survey which measures participants at one point in time and may entail comparing between subgroups of the people surveyed. It would be sensible in the Discussion to acknowledge that a causal chain of events cannot be established as all of the variables will have been measured at one time. When looking at the Method part of the report, you will need to see whether the 'gold standard' design – the randomised controlled trial – has been deployed to minimise a risk of bias among participants and researchers by making them both 'blind' to which participants are randomly allocated into the control and experimental groups. What you will need to be vigilant in spotting

---

[1] Remember that significance level refers to the pre-specified level that researchers set when determining whether the results they have obtained are due merely to chance (see Chapter 6).

is the presence of potential **extraneous variables** (that is, variables external to the participants such as extremes of noise or heat) or **confounding variables** that are specific to the individual participants. A typical confounding variable would be a personality trait, such as anger-proneness, which has been implicated in risk of coronary heart disease (CHD) (Booth-Kewley and Friedman, 1987) but which may be impervious to manipulation by a researcher studying the pharmacological effects of a beta-blocker drug for preventing CHD.

Sampling

When looking at how well designed a study is, you need to check for the sample size. Does it look as if the authors have got a large enough sample? Remember the exercise that we covered in Chapter 4 on the importance of sizeable samples that give an optimal estimate of the population mean? Does it look as if the sample has been chosen **randomly** (for example, with a random numbers table or computer program) or with a pseudo-random strategy (for example, by picking names out of a hat)? If the sampling hasn't followed these methods, does it look as if it has been chosen in a non-biased way? How do the authors defend their use of sampling technique? Are they using a stratified approach to get sufficient proportions of people from different cross-sections of a study population? Getting a stratified sample is when the researchers set a quota of people to be sampled. This is especially important when there are small numbers of people at different levels within the population of interest. For example, you might be interested in studying the role of social class as an influencing factor for inequalities in coronary heart disease. If there are few people in the lowest and highest social classes within the population, it might be preferable to get a predefined percentage of participants (say, 10 per cent) from each social class.

As we highlighted in Chapter 4, it is important that the researchers avoid bias when selecting a sample so that, ideally, participants have an equal chance of being recruited into the study. In this way, the study results have a better likelihood of being generalisable to the wider study population.

Variables

Another series of questions you could ask when looking at the Method section relates to the types of variable that are being assessed. You should be able to find how the variables are defined on a conceptual level (that is, how the variables relate to nursing theory or practice). Moreover, you will need to know how data on these variables were gathered by looking for the quality of the tools used – this will usually be found in a 'Stimuli', 'Materials', 'Measures' or 'Equipment' subsection to the Method. You need to ask whether the tools seem appropriate for measurements into the specific research topic. For example, it may be that you are reading about a mental health nursing study and clients are being assessed with the Beck Depression Inventory (Beck *et al.*, 1988).

You could ask yourself whether this instrument is the only or best way to detect a client's risk of depression. Could other tools be used, such as the Hospital Anxiety and Depression (HAD) scale (Mykletun *et al.*, 2001)? Are you interested in a certain type of depression, such as post-natal depression? If so, it could be that the Edinburgh Postnatal Depression Scale (EPDS; Cox *et al.*, 1987) is more appropriate to the particular symptoms of depression after childbirth. You will need to ask yourself whether the researchers have justified their choice of how they collect the data. Do the researchers report any information about the validity and/or reliability of the instruments being used? With the excerpt in Box 9.1, taken from a fictionalised article looking into studying burnout among nurses, use a highlighter pen to identify any good practices with reporting on the properties of the tools used in the study.

Evaluating how variables are defined and measured

When looking at any alternative variables that could have been assessed, you will need to evaluate the content of how these variables were measured in the study. Do all of the questionnaire items or rating scales or other measures make sense to you? In other words, what is their face validity or acceptability? Do they appear to be tapping into the areas that the researchers intended to study? For instance, if you're looking at whether patients on a weight-loss programme are overweight, would you be using something like a body mass index, taking into account height and weight, or would you use other indices such as a person's hip to waist ratio? As this example illustrates, there are various ways to monitor the type of patient health or illness that you're interested in and it will be essential for the study's authors to defend why they have chosen certain variables and methods of measurement. Table 9.3 provides an overview of the types of questions that would be asked when critically appraising the design.

Table 9.3 Section 2 of the critical appraisal framework

Section	Where to look in the research report	What questions to ask
2. Design	Method	● Is there a clear statement and justification for the choice of design (e.g. randomised controlled trial vs other designs)?
		● Do the researchers attempt to minimise bias with their sampling techniques (e.g. by using random sampling)?
		● Is there an attempt to control for or consider extraneous or confounding variables?
		● Have the instruments/methods of collecting data been defended in terms of reliability and validity?
		● Are the measured variables explained and justified sufficiently?
		● Should other variables have been measured instead?

222

Box 9.1 Task

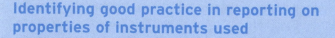

Identifying good practice in reporting on properties of instruments used

With a highlighter pen, identify the sections of this Method section that deal with defending the selection of the research instrument. What other things could have been said to justify why the instrument was used?

Materials

The research instrument used for this survey was a postal questionnaire consisting of several sections. Section A provided demographic details such as age, gender and the nurses' level of seniority. The following sections consisted of 22 items, which were the three scales from the Maslach Burnout Inventory (MBI; Maslach and Jackson, 1986), which measured emotional exhaustion (section B), personal achievement (section C) and depersonalisation (section D). Participants rated each of the items on a seven-point Likert response scale of frequency, ranging from 0 (never) to 6 (every day). The concept of emotional exhaustion has been found to measure the extent to which the nurses felt that they were unable to present positive emotions to their patients (Williams and Gregg, 1998). Personal achievement is a construct that has been found when nurses feel that their work is meaningful (Allen & Tammy, 1988); low scores on this scale would tend to symbolise a higher risk of the nurse suffering from burnout. Depersonalisation has been shown by Mcleod (1986) as being the stage whereby nurses will tend to neglect the needs and humanity of their patients. Face validity of the questionnaire was achieved by reviewing the questionnaire's format and content among qualified nurses ($n = 56$) who were not included in the main study. Reliability analysis showed that all three constructs in the questionnaire had good internal consistency, with Cronbach's alpha coefficients of, respectively, 0.85, 0.86 and 0.89. Previous studies have shown that the MBI has moderate to high levels of discriminant validity (for example, Pines and Maslach, 1988) and high levels of construct validity (Maslach and Brief, 1989).

● Section 3: Analysis

In some research papers there is a subsection in the Method section called 'Analysis'. This subsection is used to outline the statistical tests that were conducted on the data, before the results of these analyses are reported in the Results section. This is your

CHAPTER 9 ● CRITICAL APPRAISAL OF ANALYSIS AND REPORTING OF INFERENTIAL STATISTICS chance to look back at the statistics jigsaw introduced in Chapter 1. What you need to be able to identify is what sorts of data are being analysed. Have the authors got categorical-type data or continuous-type data? You need to look at the number of variables being measured as well as the type of data. In this book, we have covered the analysis of two variables of various types. If you find that the authors are analysing three or more variables, we recommend that you look at a more advanced text that covers multivariate analysis. However, this text gives you the fundamentals for performing the most basic tests that all nurse researchers need to be able to perform. By using the statistics jigsaw, which we have pieced together throughout the book, why not try assessing whether the right test has been done for each of the two case examples? Box 9.2 presents selections from two published articles. Read these and then answer the questions that follow.

Box 9.2 Task

Critically appraising the choice of statistical test and full reportage of the results from the test

Case example 1 – from Spence and El-Ansari (2004) Portfolio assessment: practice teachers' early experience

Summary

Two questionnaires sought the views of specialist community nursing practitioner programme . . . practice teachers (PTs) on the introduction of the portfolio approach to practice assessment. These were distributed to 62 and 76 PTs and the response rates were 32% and 50%, respectively. Responses of those PTs from the three specialisms participating in the piloting of the portfolio approach were compared with those using an existing approach.

In questionnaire A, one item was open ended in order to generate qualitative data. Quantitatively, this questionnaire comprised 18 items (employing 5-point Likert scales) to determine respondents' agreement or disagreement [with] a series of statements.

As the responses to most questions were not normally distributed, the Mann–Whitney U test was used to study the underlying population distributions (Gibbons and Chakraborti, 1992). Samples' responses to the questions with Likert scale results were compared across groups using the Mann–Whitney U test. The percentage of respondents reporting positively was compared using the t-test for equality of means (Black, 1999).

Questionnaire items where significant differences were noted between pilot and non-pilot respondents, together with respective means, are presented in Table 3. Pilot PTs used significantly less first-hand experience of the students' practice in their assessments and used significantly more portfolio evidence in the process.

Table 3: Sources of evidence: pilot and non-pilot groups

Source of evidence	Contribution to student assessment (mean %)		p value
	Pilot	Non-pilot	
PT use of first-hand experience of the student's practice in the assessment process	28.8	43.7	0.02
PT use of written evidence compiled in the portfolio in the assessment process	25.2	11.25	0.03

Is the method of variable measurement clear?   Yes/No

(give your reasons): _____

_____

Has the choice of statistical tests been justified?   Yes/No

(give your reasons): _____

_____

Is there sufficient information on what was found with these tests?   Yes/No

(give your reasons): _____

_____

Case example 2 – from Finlay *et al.* (1998) A randomized controlled study of portfolio learning in undergraduate cancer education [for medical students]

Method

Following a description of the project to the whole year group, students were given the opportunity to opt out of the trial. The remaining students were randomly assigned to either the study group or the control group. The study group was allocated into tutorial groups for the experimental programme, while the control group continued the standard curriculum with no extra input. The study continued until the end of the clinical course.

Method

Final assessment was by hidden questions in the final degree examination in the form of three stations in the Pharmacology and Therapeutics objective structured clinical examination (OSCE). Two stations of 4 minutes, each in a standard format, asked questions about the management of malignant intestinal obstruction and of metastatic breast cancer. The third station of 8 minutes was a role play where the student had to play the role of a surgical house officer explaining to a patient's daughter that her father had metastatic prostate cancer and needed hormonal therapy and palliative radiotherapy. Sixteen role players (13 oncology nurses and three radiographers) were trained to play the daughter and complete standard assessment forms for factual accuracy and communication skills of the students. All examination results were analysed using the t-test for two samples assuming unequal variances, including all those who had been randomized to the study vs the controls.

Results

... a total of 159 students ... were randomly allocated into the control (79) and study (80) groups.

The OSCE examination showed no significant difference between the two groups overall or for the oncology questions or role play. However, on all counts, the trend was towards a better performance by the study group.

Table: OSCE results: all students

Number of students	Mean (variance)		
	Control $n = 69$	Study $n = 68$	p
All questions (expressed as % of 128 marks)	50.2 (25)	50.4 (18)	n.s.
Oncology and role play (maximum possible mark = 12)	11.1 (4)	11.5 (3)	n.s.
Oncology questions (maximum possible mark = 8)	5.9 (1.1)	6.2 (0.7)	0.06
Role play (maximum possible mark = 4)	2.5 (0.7)	2.7 (0.6)	n.s.

Is the method of variable measurement clear?   Yes/No

(give your reasons): _____

_____

Has the choice of statistical tests been justified?   Yes/No

(give your reasons): _____

_____

Is there sufficient information on what was found with these tests?   Yes/No

(give your reasons): _____

_____

Sources: Case example 1 – excerpts from W. Spence, and W. El-Ansari (2004) 'Portfolio assessment: practice teachers' early experience', Nurse Education Today, *24: 388–401. Reproduced with permission of Elsevier Science. Case example 2 – excerpts from I.G. Finlay, T.S. Maughan and D.J. Webster (1998) 'A randomized controlled study of portfolio learning in undergraduate cancer education',* Medical Education, *32: 172–176.*

Table 9.4 Section 3 of the critical appraisal framework

Section	Where to look in the research report	What questions to ask
3. Analysis	Method and Results	● What sorts of data are being analysed? ● Does the performed test fit with the type of data obtained? ● Could alternative statistical tests have been done on the data?

Table 9.4 summarises the sorts of question that you will have been asking for section 3 of the critical appraisal framework regarding the analysis strategies outlined by authors in the Method section of a paper.

● Section 4: Reporting findings

When critically appraising how the results are reported, one simple thing to do before looking at the inferential statistics is to spot any reporting of the descriptive statistics. You will have covered critically appraising descriptive statistics in Chapter 5, but it should mainly suffice at this stage to see whether the authors have provided an overall picture of the data by reporting the summaries, such as means, standard deviations and whether some variables correlate with each other in a correlation matrix. Another superficial check, but important nonetheless, is to do a spot check of any statistics used to make inferences about whether the data obtained are significantly different from what would be obtained by chance. Is there mention of the degrees of freedom and sample size for each analysis? Is the significance level reported as well? Is the type of test indicated through the use of a symbol (such as a *t* indicating that a *t*-test statistic has been generated)? As practice in carrying out the spot checks of the important features to be included in any inferential statistical analyses, try the exercise in Box 9.3.

Box 9.3 Task

Identifying sample size, levels of significance and other vital statistics

The following are excerpts from studies into healthcare organisation and nursing. To what extent do the results presented give the main inferential statistics on sample size, significance and other important areas? Use these five questions for each of the tables or descriptions of the results:

1. What is the test that has been conducted?

2. What is the sample size?

3. What are the degrees of freedom for this test?

4. What is the level of significance for the test?

5. Is the statistic significant?

Excerpt 1 – from Nairn *et al.* (2006)

Table: Analysis by year of study for students' knowledge of systems of portfolio use and attitudes towards its utility

Questionnaire item	Year of study	Means (S.D.)	*t*-test analysis
'I know I should show my portfolio to my mentor during my placement'	First/Second Third/Fourth	2.71 (1.42) 1.91 (1.04)	$p = 0.00$ $t = 6.20$ $d.f. = 381.25$ $n = 386$

Excerpt 2 – from Nairn *et al.* (2006)

There was a significant relationship between year on course and perceptions of becoming better at using portfolios ($p = 0.00$; $\chi^2 = 76.4$; $d.f. = 2$; $n = 353$).

▶ ### Excerpt 3 – from fictionalised article by Williams and Maltby (2010)

Additionally, the more anxious patients became, the less information that they were able to remember when given pre-operative instructions on dealing with post-operative pain ($r = -0.179$, $n = 174$, $p = 0.036$).

Source: Excerpts 1 and 2 from S. Nairn, E. O'Brien, V. Traynor, G. Williams, M. Chapple and S. Johnson (2006). 'Student nurses' knowledge, skills and attitudes towards the use of portfolios in a school of nursing', Journal of Clinical Nursing, *in press.*

Clear data reporting

The other key elements to look for when critically appraising the reporting of inferential statistics is whether the authors have clearly expressed the main trends when making sense of the statistics. What not to do would be something like this:

> A significant main effect was found for type of healthcare team and team objective setting.

If this is all that the authors tell you, then they haven't provided enough information to make sense of the data. All that the authors seem to be saying is that the type of healthcare team has some influence on how the team sets its objectives. This isn't really that helpful as we don't know what teams are involved or the extent to which some teams are better at setting their team objectives than are others. The following sentence shows a clearer illustration of what the main trends are and how the authors made sense of the results:

A further independent-groups t-test revealed that multidisciplinary clinic teams (M = 22.87) scored statistically significantly more highly than primary health care teams (M = 9.74) in terms of team objective setting.

(Williams and Laungani, 1999, p. 24)

What you're looking for is clarity in expressing the identified differences or relationships for a specified variable and whether the authors have shown the direction of differences or strength of the relationships as well. As an overview, the types of question posed when critically appraising the reporting of the data are covered in Table 9.5.

There is sometimes an area of ambiguity regarding how to comment on the results. Basically, it should be remembered that the authors need simply report the main trends and give no speculations as to the reasons for the results in the Results section. Any attempts at interpreting the results and making sense of why these results were obtained should be confined to the Discussion section.

Table 9.5 Section 4 of the critical appraisal framework

Section	Where to look in the research report	What questions to ask
4. Reporting findings	Results	● Is there a description of the overall picture of the data (e.g. means and standard deviations)?
		● When reporting inferential statistics, is there mention of degrees of freedom, sample size, the test statistic and significance level?
		● Is there a clear expression of the observed differences or relationships between variables and what these differences/relationships means?

● Section 5: Interpretation and contextualisation of findings

In the Discussion section, you should be looking for the authors to provide a brief summary of the findings – this is not for the authors to repeat the statistics mentioned in the Results section or to come up with findings not already covered in the Results. It is also a chance for the authors to give their interpretations of why certain trends were obtained. For example, if non-significant findings were obtained there should be some analysis as to why this was the case. Also, the authors will get no prizes for highlighting only significant results that support their viewpoint. Although nursing research papers are essentially arguments for going in a specific direction in terms of research, theory or practice, the authors should still entertain alternative explanations for the data they have collected. Also, when reading the Discussion, ask yourself whether the authors are speculating beyond the results obtained. For example, are they arguing for using multi-layered dressings for all patients with leg ulcers when it has been found effective only with one type of leg ulcer?

Contextualising findings in line with the Introduction

Another element that a good Discussion should have is that it should clearly define whether data confirm or disconfirm the hypotheses set out in the Introduction. If a hypothesis cannot be retained, do the authors attempt to generate **alternative hypotheses** for further research? As many good researchers will recognise, the process for doing research is an ongoing one, whereby data often throw up more questions than answers, leading to deciding on possible directions for conducting further research. Therefore it is essential for the authors to provide suggestions for future studies in the area. Excellent recommendations go beyond simple ideas of getting larger samples (although sometimes this helps when the original study involves analysis of data for a sample of just 20 or so participants). The better research reports entail proposals for more effective designs and alternative methods of analysis. The astute authors will cover limitations of their study to pre-empt the kinds of concerns that readers might have over the data collected. Most importantly, you need to check whether the authors make explicit attempts to make sense of their data in light of healthcare policies and clinical practice procedures. The Discussion needs to show that the nursing theory and research have preceded the generation of hypotheses in the study and that the authors aren't quoting any new research not covered in the Introduction. If the studies were that important, they should have been mentioned in the Introduction. The crucial thing with critical appraisal is that you recognise that everything has its place and that readers will be looking for research conducted prior to the study only in the Introduction.

Making an overall summary of the study's quality

Finally, although we have not dedicated a special section in the critical appraisal framework to this area, it will be helpful to make an overall assessment of how good the paper is. List the general strengths and limitations of the study and see whether you can

Table 9.6 Section 5 and general observations section of the critical appraisal framework

Section	Where to look in the research report	What questions to ask
5. Interpretation and contextualisation of findings	Discussion	● At the start of the Discussion, is there a brief summary of the findings? ● Is there a statement as to whether the hypotheses have been rejected or retained? Are alternative hypotheses entertained? ● Are there attempts to give explanations for the results obtained? ● Is there an acknowledgement of alternative interpretations of the results? ● Is there a clear link between the results and the implications for practice/further research, or is there speculation beyond what has been found? ● Is there a coherent plan for further research to expand upon the findings obtained? ● Is the study related to developments in research, healthcare policy or nursing practice? ● Are new studies introduced in the Discussion, rather than in the Introduction?
General observations	All sections, including Abstract	● What are the overall strengths of the study? ● What are the study's limitations? ● Is the study's main message apparent and is it revisited throughout the report?

summarise the main message that the authors are trying to convey. Is the study's message apparent from reading the Abstract? Do the authors keep revisiting this main message throughout the paper or do they depart from the main point from time to time? One way to get to the gist of the study is to look for concepts that are repeated during the paper. Overall, use of our critical appraisal framework should help you to assess, at a glance, the quality of the research and how well it is reported. An overview of the questions to ask in section 5 of the critical appraisal framework and looking at the overall quality of the paper is provided in Table 9.6.

Applying the critical appraisal framework

Using the critical appraisal framework, ask searching questions about the quality of the design, analysis and reporting of the fictionalised case study in Box 9.4, which uses data from the adult branch dataset. Although fictitious, the case study is typical of articles that you will encounter in nursing journals.

Fictionalised case study article for use with the critical appraisal framework

ASSESSMENT OF NUTRITIONAL PROBLEMS AND RISK OF FALLING IN HOSPITAL-BASED OLDER PERSON CARE: BRIEF RESEARCH REPORT

F. Ward, G.A. Williams, J. Maltby and L. Day

Abstract

Falls among older people are problematic in the hospital environment and a cause for concern among administrators, patients, relatives and health professionals alike. In the current study, the views of 31 nurses on falls' risk assessment were obtained from a randomly selected sample of 50 nursing staff working in three care of the older person wards. We focused on nurses' consideration of poor nutrition among patients as being a major factor for making falls more likely and hypothesised that there would be a relationship between the type of ward that a nurse was based on and acknowledging nutritional problems as being implicated with falls. No significant link was found between ward type and nurses looking at nutrition. We outline the implications for staff training with needing to ensure that more nurses see nutrition as a falls' risk factor. It is also recommended that this education does not need to target those working in only one type of care of the older person ward.

Box 9.4 Study

Introduction

Falls among older people contribute greatly to mortality and morbidity throughout this country and the government (Department of Health and Health Care, 2003) has been implementing action plans to target this growing problem. The Dietetic Society (2007) has claimed that one of the major risk factors for falls among older people is that many of them are undernourished, thus leading to dizziness when older people are mobilising. In the hospital environment, there should be less chance of older patients not having sufficient nourishment, as there should be more control over what food is administered to them. However, there is evidence that the older patient has problems with diet and feeling hungry due to polypharmacy (i.e. needing to take a cocktail of prescribed drugs throughout the day) (Jefferies and Dealer, 2006). In the current study, we were aiming to see whether nurses involved with care of the older patient were taking poor diet/malnourishment into account when considering a patient's risk of falling. This study focused on the reported falls' risk assessment practices of a sample of registered general nurses working at three care of the older person wards in a community hospital based in a city within the New Pleasant state. We also sought to explore whether there was a relationship between the type of ward that the nurses worked on and the reported assessment practices. It was hypothesised that there would be a link between ward and assessment of diet when examining risk of falling. This hypothesis was grounded in observations by the research team that one of the wards (Spondlebury) appeared to have patients with higher dependencies than in the other two wards, which dealt mainly with rehabilitation, and that staff would thus have less time to consider nutrition as an issue.

Method

Participants

A random sample of 50 nurses was approached out of the population of 75 full-time and part-time nurses employed by the hospital. Agency nursing staff was not approached, as the permanent staff would govern all induction and training in patient assessment and we viewed them as being vital to driving the methods and ethos of patient assessment. Out of the nurses that we sampled, 33 replied to the invitation letter with a completed questionnaire (66 per cent response rate), although only 31 of the forms were useable with complete data.

Materials

We used the Stanislav Falls Assessment Procedures Index (Stanislav, 2005). This comprised a 35-item form that requires respondents to identify the factors they consider when assessing an older person's risk of falling. This questionnaire has been mainly validated with hospital-based older person care (Stanislav and Spector, 2004) and has been found to have subscales tapping into three main concepts: physical health, psychological well-being and the mobilisation process. These three subscales have internal consistencies of 0.89, 0.65 and 0.85 respectively.

Analysis

As we were primarily interested in the relationship between type of care of the older person ward and nurses' reported assessment of nutritional problems when examining patient risk of falling, we conducted a chi-square analysis on these two variables.

Procedure

Posters advertising the study were placed on staff noticeboards near the three wards and the agreement of the staff unions and the hospital management was obtained before commencing the study. Local Research Ethical Committee approval was also granted in November 2005. The research team sent the questionnaire to the sample of nurses via the internal post during the week commencing 12 December 2005. The forms had a self-addressed, stamped envelope for participants to send their completed returns to the team by a two-week deadline.

Results

Table 1 outlines the distribution of nurses who said that they either did or did not consider nutritional problems among their patients when assessing risk of falling on the wards. It is noteworthy that only 16 out of the 31 (51.6 per cent) nurse respondents reported looking out for nutritional problems when assessing falls' risk.

Table 1: Nutritional problems as a risk factor for falls among older patients

'Which ward do you work in?'	'Consideration of nutrition problems?'	
	No	Yes
Spondlebury	5	6
Wickham	7	7
Hesham	3	3

A chi-square analysis showed that there was no significant relationship between the type of ward that the nurses worked on and their focus on nutritional problems among patients when conducting falls' risk assessment, $\chi^2(2) = 0.059$, $p > 0.05$.

Discussion

It can be seen from the results that only half of the nurses who responded to our survey of falls' risk assessment practices said that they considered nutritional problems among their patients. This trend is in line with prior research (for example, William and Hill, 2003) showing that nutrition is a neglected part of inpatient care for the older person and that nutritional well-being tends to be left to the dietician to monitor (Tidy and Meal, 2000). Unexpectedly, there was no link between type of ward and evaluation of nutritional problems as a risk factor, thus indicating that nursing practice seems fairly consistent within a community hospital setting.

There are some potential limitations that need to be considered. Although our sample of 31 respondents was a sizeable percentage of the population of nursing staff within the three wards, it needs to be recognised that there may have been fewer senior nurses obtained with random sampling as they constitute a relatively small percentage of the total number of nurses employed in the study sites. Given that it is likely the senior nurses would be more involved with patient assessment (and falls' risk assessment) than junior nurses, this could explain why only half of our sample had considered nutrition as a factor. Further research could aim at replicating the administration of our questionnaire to staff at other similar wards, but through the use of a stratified sampling method. Nevertheless, the current trends seem to suggest the need for nursing practice to routinely incorporate the nutritional status of an older patient and for nurses to be educated about the impact that poor nutrition among older patients can have on making the patient disorientated and weak when mobilising. As we did not find a link between type of care of the older person ward and reported assessment practices, we would recommend that this education should cover the training of all grades of nursing and in all types of wards.

Exercise

Apply the critical appraisal framework from this chapter to the above study by using the following section headings:

Section 1: Hypotheses and significance levels

....

....

....

....

Section 2: Design

....

....

....

....

Section 3: Analysis

....

....

....

Section 4: Reporting findings

....

....

....

Section 5: Interpretation and contextualisation of findings

....

....

....

General observations

....

....

....

By using the critical appraisal framework, you should now have a clear understanding of the strengths and limitations of the study that you have just critically appraised. You can find some of our own suggestions for the critical appraisal of this study by going to the book's website at www.pearsoned.co.uk/maltby.

Summary

In this chapter, we have:

✔ introduced you to a critical appraisal framework for examining the quality of a research report or journal article under five main headings: (1) hypotheses/ significance testing, (2) design, (3) analysis, (4) reporting and (5) contextualisation and interpretation;

✔ enabled you to apply the critical appraisal framework to a fictitious article in order to analyse the rigorousness of the reporting of inferential statistical analyses.

In the following chapter we will point you towards advancing your knowledge of statistics by introducing the notion of clinical significance and deciding on appropriate sample sizes for studies that you do in the future. You can also use the ideas on clinical and statistical significance to decide whether to integrate research findings into your everyday clinical practice.

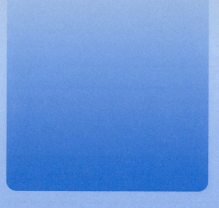

Chapter 10

Advanced thinking with probability and significance: where to next?

Key themes

- ✔ Statistical significance
- ✔ Clinical/practical significance
- ✔ Effect size
- ✔ Percentage improvement
- ✔ Probability
- ✔ Hypothesis testing
- ✔ Error
- ✔ Confidence intervals

Learning outcomes

By the end of this chapter you will be able to outline ideas of:

- ✔ Statistical and clinical significance, and how these relate to effect size and percentage improvement in a research participant's condition
- ✔ Hypothesis testing and confidence intervals, and how these two concepts are used in the literature to provide context (frameworks) to statistical findings

Introduction

Imagine . . . That you are a mental health nurse who has been tasked with finding journal articles that show the effectiveness (or lack of effectiveness) of a new drug used to treat psychotic symptoms with clients who have schizophrenia. Your charge nurse has given you the job of informing the rest of the mental healthcare team about the evidence base for this drug and whether the team should adopt the drug as the treatment of choice. You have now reviewed the literature and found three articles that have reported the use of this medication with samples of no more than 100 clients in each study. The problem is that none of these studies has shown a statistically significant improvement in the psychotic symptoms of clients with schizophrenia when comparing before and after administration of the drug. There have also not been statistically significant differences between groups of clients who have taken the drug and those who have not. However, there are indications that the clients have fewer psychotic symptoms and fewer side effects when taking the medication; it's just that the effects found are not statistically significant. By using these statistical trends, it would be likely that you could only propose that your team does not adopt the drug as treatment of choice for schizophrenia. What makes the decision even more complicated is that there is a concept known as 'clinical significance'. On a practical level, if you are finding that your clients are improving and having fewer side effects with the medication, it might still be worthwhile to recommend the drug if it can be concluded that the drug will make life more pleasant and symptom-free for your clients. We will be looking at the distinction between clinical and statistical significance later in this chapter.

Throughout the book we have introduced you to a number of statistical tests, and have shown you how results from these tests help us to establish whether relationships or differences between two variables are statistically significant. However, in this last chapter we are going to introduce you to a number of terms that represent advanced statistical testing about how statisticians report and use probability. We need to do this because researchers in the nursing literature often use many of the newer terms and procedures that we will be covering in this chapter and we want to bring you as up to date as possible. We're not going to emphasise some of the statistical procedures that surround these ideas, because they are advanced statistical ideas and are often used in the design of research studies or research methods, or reflect judgements that relate to statistics in the real world. Therefore, we are going to highlight how, when and where these ideas are used around reporting of statistics so that when you come across them in the nursing literature you are not confused or thrown off by the mention of them.

Therefore in this chapter we are going to extend on some of the ideas we have covered in the preceding chapters. The extension of these ideas is not designed to confuse you or to say you should do something different; you can see them as add-ons which can increase your statistical knowledge. Remember how we added on the idea of effect size to correlations (and other statistical tests) to help you say whether statistical findings have a small (0.2), medium (0.5) or large (0.8) effect? That was fairly straightforward and easy to remember, and you should treat what we introduce in this chapter in a similar way. These are statistical procedures which help you make accurate judgements about your data.

We have divided these considerations into two main areas, but they are, like many other statistical procedures, related. These two areas are: (1) statistical and clinical significance and (2) hypothesis testing and confidence intervals. Therefore at the end of this chapter you should be able to outline ideas that underlie statistical and clinical significance and how these relate to effect size and percentage improvement in a research participant's condition. You will also be able to outline the ideas that form hypothesis testing and confidence intervals, and how these two concepts are used in the literature to provide context to statistical findings.

Statistical versus clinical significance

Within the statistical literature there is a distinction between **statistical significance** and **clinical significance**. Throughout this book we have concentrated on reporting statistical significance because these are changes that are primarily related to the use of statistical tests. However, when we report the findings from statistical tests, a number of questions can arise about the practical importance of these findings. These questions are best summarised by the one question: are findings clinically (or practically) significant?

Let us frame this distinction with the following examples. Researchers might have found that a drug treatment has had a statistically significant effect on a particular illness. To do this, doctors and researchers would have administered the drug to different groups and looked at changes in the symptoms of the illness of individuals in all groups. These groups usually include:

- **Experimental groups** – groups that receive an intervention (for example, a drug, a counselling session).
- **Control groups** – groups that do not receive an intervention but are used to compare the extent of effects with the experimental group. For example, in a drug trial, some individuals will receive a placebo, a substance containing no medication, which acts as a control (or comparison) condition.

However, they would have been particularly interested in reporting whether there was a statistically significant change in symptoms (in other words, patients in the experimental groups showing statistically significantly fewer symptoms of the illness) as a result of the use of the new drug. However, various people (nurses, patients, doctors, patients' relatives) might wonder whether, notwithstanding that the drug has been found to have a statistically significant effect, it has a clinically (or practical) significant effect. For example, does the administration of the drug lead to a clinically significant improvement in the patients' lives? For example, although the drug has been found to have an effect on certain aspects of the illness (perhaps inflammation or serum level), the patient might be concerned whether it will lead to improved sense of well-being or even to a longer life. Healthcare professionals would also be concerned whether the drug would be of clinical significance for a group of people that they are treating for a particular illness. For example, if the doctor is going to start using a new drug, will this drug be considered to have enough of a clinical significance effect to generally be found to work among a number of patients, particularly when considered alongside a number of available treatments?

Equally, people might consider using something that has clinical significance even when that something isn't statistically significant. For example, the new drug might not have been found to lead to a statistically significant difference in the groups who received the drug, but nonetheless a number of patients might have shown a clinical change in symptoms. Therefore, the drug will still be of interest to people because it has brought about beneficial changes in some patients, and, particularly where there is a lack of alternative treatments, people might consider investigating the use of the drug further.

Therefore, clinical significance has little to do with statistics, but rather it is a judgement. It considers the idea of whether relationships or differences between two variables are of a certain significance even if they are or are not statistically significant. Remember, findings from studies can be statistically significant yet clinically non-significant. Conversely, findings from studies might be statistically non-significant yet clinically significant.

However, statisticians have usefully provided us with some statistical procedures to guide our thinking around these issues. It is important to stress that these statistics are all judgements and questions that surround a particular area. These do not comprise absolute criteria, as we had with statistical tests, by which we could decide whether something was statistically significant or not. There are no right or wrong answers with these statistics, and they should be used only to inform your thinking and guide your judgements regarding clinical significance. We cannot stress this strongly enough. Your final judgements will be based not only these statistics but also on what you are studying, the research area, the literature and what other people (mentors supervising student nurse placements, your lecturers and other nursing colleagues) suggest.

The two statistics that might guide us in our judgements about clinical significance are:

- effect size;
- percentage improvement.

● Effect size

The effect size is the most commonly used method of assessing clinical significance. We have already introduced you to effect size in Chapter 7 on correlations and Chapter 8 on statistics that compare differences between groups and occasions. However, to act as a reminder we will briefly go through the same points again, and produce some of the statistics and calculations that are required particularly within the context of experimental and control groups.

Effect size simply refers to the strength of the relationship. Luckily the criteria of 0.2 (small), 0.5 (medium) and 0.8 (large) introduced by statistician Jacob Cohen (1988) to label the effect size are used across the majority of the statistics mentioned (though it won't surprise you that practice varies, but to a lesser extent than other areas of statistics). Cohen suggested that effect sizes of 0.2 to 0.5 should be regarded as small, 0.5 to 0.8 as moderate and above 0.8 as large. Therefore an effect size of

- 0.2 represents a *small* effect size;
- 0.5 represents a *medium* (or *moderate*) effect size;
- 0.8 represents a *large* effect size.

It is best to see these criteria as set out in Table 10.1.

With correlation statistics (for example, Pearson and Spearman correlation) effect size can be determined from the size of the correlation statistic. So, for example, a finding in which the correlation statistic (*r* or *rho*) is 0.2 would be considered as having a small clinical significance, whereas a finding in which the correlation statistic is 0.8 would have large clinical significance. (For more information on this, read the effect size section in Chapter 7.)

With tests of difference (for example, independent-samples *t*-test and paired-samples *t*-test), the effect size (*d*) for differences between two sets of scores is calculated using the statistical formula $d = M_1 - M_2 / \sigma$. This actually means:

Table 10.1 Cohen's effect size criteria

Criteria	Effect size
	1.0
	0.9
Large	0.8
↑	0.7
	0.6
Medium/moderate	0.5
↑	0.4
	0.3
Small	0.2
	0.1
	0.0

$$\text{Effect size} = \frac{\text{Mean of first group of scores} - \text{Mean of second group of scores}}{\text{Standard deviation of all scores } (\sigma)}$$

To read more on this, with examples, go back to Chapter 8.

However, there is one more effect size that we haven't covered that is used when we are considering the effect size of differences between groups. The reason we are going to highlight this is because it refers to occasions when there is an experimental group and a control group and therefore you may come across this in the nursing and medical literature, particularly when researchers are testing drugs. It is slightly different from the calculation above but nonetheless we thought we would point it out so you didn't get confused. When you have an experimental group and control group, the way that effect size is worked out is to

subtract the **control group mean** (M_2) from the **experimental group mean** (M_1) and divide that by the **standard deviation of scores of the control group** (σ_2)

The statistical formula is $d = (M_1 - M_2) / \sigma_2$. This will give you the clinical significance of differences between experimental and control groups.

There is one final point which we have raised before in this book but is worth repeating here. These considerations are about judgement and it is always worth considering from a nursing/medical perspective the clinical significance of small effect sizes. Robert Rosenthal (1991) has pointed out that the importance of effect sizes may depend on the sort of question we are investigating. For example, finding a small correlation between emergency ward volume and time spent at patients' bedsides might suggest that there isn't an important effect on emergency ward volume and the amount of bed-side care. However, when it comes to aspects such as medication, if there is a small effect size between a new drug and its ability to save lives suggesting that it saves 4 out 100 lives, then translating that figure to a population of 100,000 would mean that 4,000 lives could be saved. This finding is certainly an important effect, regardless of the effect size.

● Percentage improvement

A second way that is used to assess clinical significance is to examine percentage improvement. Percentage improvement is used in situations where the researcher is comparing differences between groups or occasions; for example, when you are looking at before and after effects of a drug intervention or when you are comparing experimental and control groups. In these situations the researcher assesses the percentage improvement that has occurred as a result of any intervention or comparison. So, for example, if we are administering a new drug, what percentage improvement among our sample does that lead to? A convention in statistics is that a *25 per cent improvement or greater* represents a clinically significant difference.

To work out a percentage improvement for before and after conditions, the calculation is:

Percentage improvement

$$= \frac{\text{(Group mean before intervention} - \text{Group mean after intervention)}}{\text{Group mean before intervention}} \times 100$$

That is, you subtract the mean for the group after the intervention from the mean for the group before the intervention. You then divide that number by the mean for the group before the intervention. You then multiple that number by 100. This gives you the percentage improvement.

As an example, suppose the mean number of symptoms for an illness group of 20 people was 10.0 before a drug trial, and after the drug trial the mean number of symptoms for the same people was 5.0. We would then subtract 5 (the mean for the group after the intervention) from 10 (the mean for the group before the intervention), which = 5. We would then divide this by the mean for the group before the intervention which is 5. So 5 divided by 5 is 1. We would then multiple this by 100; 1 multiplied by 100 is 100, and expressed as a percentage is 100 per cent. Therefore with the present group the percentage improvement of this drug is 100 per cent. This is above the '25 per cent improvement or greater' criterion and represents a clinically significant difference.

Furthermore, in studies in which there is an intervention group *and* a control group you can assess the percentage improvement of the use of the drug by taking into account any percentage improvement with the control group. Let us say, for example, that our intervention group (as above) had shown a percentage improvement of 100 per cent. Let us also say we had run a control group as well, and the percentage improvement for the control group had been 20 per cent.

Percentage improvement
= Intervention group percentage improvement – Control group percentage improvement

So in the case of our drug above, when considering control group trials, we would subtract 20 per cent (control group percentage improvement) from 100 per cent (intervention group percentage improvement) = 80 per cent. So in this case we would be able to say that the drug led to an 80 per cent improvement among patients in the intervention group.

Hypothesis testing versus confidence intervals

We are introducing you to hypothesis testing and confidence intervals because they are formal procedures that are often used in the nursing literature to frame and aid the reporting of statistics. We won't go into too much detail here because the two procedures are largely linked to research design and methods; nonetheless we will give you enough of an introduction so that when you come across these terms in the literature you are not confused or put off by them.

Hypothesis testing

So far in this book we have looked at statistics as a way of answering research questions. However, one thing you have to be aware of is that sometimes a research question is referred to as a hypothesis. Using hypotheses is the same as using questions. However, there is some formal terminology associated with using hypotheses to describe the type of research question proposed.

In using hypotheses, you are asked to state *formally* the outcomes expected in the research, in terms of a relationship or difference between variables measured and whether you expect the results to be statistically significant. The first formal statement of outcomes relates to making a **null hypothesis**. With the null hypothesis you are suggesting that there will be *no* statistically significant relationship or difference between the variables you are measuring.

As an example, Koppers *et al.* (2006) looked at the relationship between respiratory muscle training at home (this involved a tube connected to a mouthpiece increasing dead space and prompting rebreathing of exhaled carbon dioxide) and lung function in patients with chronic obstructive pulmonary disease (COPD). COPD encompasses both chronic bronchitis and emphysema and is one of the commonest respiratory conditions of adults in the developed world. The null hypothesis for this study would be that there would be no statistically significant relationship between respiratory muscle training at home and lung function in patients with COPD.

The second statement is concerned with an **alternative hypothesis**. With the alternative hypothesis you are suggesting that there *will* be a statistically significant relationship among the variables you are measuring. Therefore, for Koppers *et al.*'s study, the alternative hypothesis would be that there would be a statistically significant relationship between respiratory muscle training at home and lung function in patients with COPD.

Finally within this area you may come across the concepts of Type I and Type II errors. **Type I** and **Type II errors** refer to the way in which researchers can classify the errors that are possible when drawing conclusions from their results using significance testing.

Remember, all inferential statistical tests are open to error because we can never be entirely sure that our sample is representative of the population from which it is drawn. Therefore we are never 100 per cent sure that our findings are correct. This is why we use significance testing, because we present our findings in terms of confidence: for example, we are 95 per cent sure ($p < 0.05$) or 99 per cent sure ($p < 0.01$). Koppers *et al.* examined 36 patients with moderate to severe COPD. Now these 36 patients are not the entire population of individuals with moderate to severe COPD so, although

Box 10.1 Point to consider

One- and two-tailed hypothesis testing

While null and alternative hypotheses involve making statements about whether there is a significant relationship (alternative hypothesis) or non-significant relationship (null hypothesis) between two variables, one-tailed and two-tailed tests involve making statements regarding the expected direction of any expected statistically significant relationship between the two variables you are measuring in the alternative hypothesis. With a one-tailed hypothesis the researcher would make a statement regarding the specific direction of the relationship. With a two-tailed hypothesis no statement is made regarding the expected relationship. So, for example, in Koppers *et al.*'s study:

- A one-tailed hypothesis would be that there would be a statistically significant *positive* relationship between respiratory muscle training at home and lung function in patients with COPD. Here the researchers are making a prediction that the relationship between respiratory muscle training at home and lung function in patients with COPD will be positive (in other words, that the more adherence to respiratory muscle training, the better the lung function).

- A two-tailed hypothesis would be that there would be a statistically significant relationship between respiratory muscle training at home and lung function in patients with COPD. Here the researchers are making no prediction about the relationship (for example, the more adherence to respiratory muscle training, the worse the lung function, or vice versa, or there is no relationship at all).

Koppers *et al.* can be confident of their findings, they can never be certain, and there is a chance they could be wrong. For example, if they used the 95 per cent confidence level ($p < 0.05$), then there is a 5 per cent chance they are wrong.

Therefore, because we are never 100 per cent sure of our results, whenever we find there is a statistically significant relationship or difference between two variables we may be wrong. Equally, when we find there is not a statistically significant relationship or difference between two variables we may also be wrong. Type I and Type II errors are used to describe the possibilities of our being wrong. Simply put, Type I error refers to an occasion when a researcher concludes that the findings are statistically significant when in actuality the findings are not significant. A Type II error refers to an occasion when a researcher concludes that the findings are not significant when in reality the findings are statistically significant.

In terms of Koppers *et al*.'s study, if they found among their sample that there was a statistically significant relationship between respiratory muscle training at home and lung function in patients with COPD, but it was later considered (through there being a study of a larger sample or a series of studies) that there was not a relationship, then this would be an example of a Type I error. However, if Koppers *et al*. found among their sample that there was *not* a statistically significant relationship between respiratory muscle training at home and lung function in patients with COPD, but it was later considered (through there being a larger sample study, or a series of studies, or a population study) that there was a statistically significant relationship, then this would be an example of a Type II error.

The possibility of making these types of error is in the minds of researchers and statisticians, and this is reflected in the language they use when considering null or alternative hypotheses in studies. It is not a major academic sin to make a Type I or Type II error (as you are always following established procedures when using statistics) and therefore it is not something you should be fearful of, or critical of, if it occurs. Rather, it is a useful way of reminding researchers that, regardless of their findings, there is always a chance that there is an error in them.

If you want to read more on hypothesis testing, refer to Box 10.1. We will see in the next section that statisticians have extended the idea of confidence and error.

● Confidence intervals

Spurred on by such concerns regarding significance levels and making Type I and Type II errors, statisticians have come up with other ways for people to state their confidence in their findings, and provide people with a more detailed account of the possible error they can make. One way of doing this that appears in the nursing literature is that of **confidence intervals**.

The best way to describe confidence intervals is by way of example. You will have come across times when organisations such as MORI (Market and Opinion Research International) have carried out an opinion poll. The government may be in crisis or there may be a general election and MORI carries out a poll in which they ask a sample of UK citizens their views on the government or who they think will win the general election. Findings from such polls usually make it on to the television news or are reported in newspapers, in which it will be stated, for example, that 56 per cent of people surveyed believe the prime minister should resign or that this political party is ahead in the polls with 42 per cent of the vote.

If you look closely at these reports (particularly in newspapers) you will see a statement next to the poll results that says something like: 'MORI interviewed a sample of 1,000, margin of error ±3%'. What this statement is saying is that, whatever conclusion the poll has presented (for example, that 56 per cent of people surveyed believe the

Table 10.2 Confidence intervals that accompany sample size at the 95 per cent probability level

Survey sample size	Confidence interval at the 95% probability level
2,000	2
1,000	3
800	3
600	4
400	5
200	7
100	10
50	14

prime minister should resign), because the poll has used a sample of people there is a margin of error (in this case, plus or minus 3 per cent) around the value presented. So the actual figure of people who believe the prime minister should resign may be as low as 53 per cent (−3 per cent) or as high as 59 per cent (+3 per cent).

Margin of error is commonly used and reported in these types of study. In nursing (and other medical disciplines) it is known as the confidence interval. It is a way of reporting the significance of our results as well as our confidence intervals (margins of error).

Confidence intervals are dependent on two things: (1) the size of the sample and (2) the probability level used to decide whether a finding is significant. Luckily for us, the 95 per cent confidence level ($p = 0.05$) is very commonly used, so that makes the other consideration relatively straightforward – that is, confidence intervals are dependent on the size of sample. Table 10.2 shows a table of the confidence intervals that accompany sample size at the 95 per cent probability level.

You can see from this table that your confidence intervals lower as your sample gets larger. The lower your confidence interval, the more you can rely on the findings. The wider the interval, the less you can rely on the findings. Therefore, a very small sample, such as 100 respondents, has a confidence interval of 10 per cent whereas a sample of 800 respondents has a confidence interval of 3 per cent.

Therefore, reporting of confidence intervals in addition to significance testing allows you as a researcher to provide even more information about your findings. The confidence interval is often described as quantifying the possible error surrounding the findings. It also allows researchers to compare findings by looking at the confidence intervals reported in different studies investigating the same or similar variables.

You will find in the nursing research literature that confidence intervals are used with many statistics. For example, you will see confidence intervals used to summarise percentage improvement or with the reporting of statistical differences in means in statistical tests (for example, the independent-samples t-test and paired-samples t-test).

To show this in terms of percentage improvement, let us take our example of percentage improvement discussed earlier in the chapter. Let us say we were trialling a new drug and we found, on average, 40 per cent improvement among 400 individuals with a confidence interval of 5 per cent (that is, ranging from 35 to 45 per cent improvement). Suppose another drug was introduced and that drug showed, on average, a 40 per cent improvement with a confidence interval of 2 per cent among 2,000 people (that is, ranging from 38 to 42 per cent improvement). With this additional information of confidence intervals we are able to quantify the possible error around the percentage improvement. Both drugs show clinical significance (that is, above 25 per cent improvement), and even though both drugs are found to show, on average, a 40 per cent improvement, you might favour the second drug because the confidence interval is less.

In terms of the reporting of statistical differences in means in statistical tests, let us revisit our finding for the independent-samples *t*-test that we covered in Chapter 8. We performed this analysis for the data in the learning disability dataset for 24 people. We looked at the relationship between two of the variables in this dataset, such as the sex of the person with the learning disability and the number of consultations that that person had had with the learning disability nurse. The independent-samples *t*-test allows the researcher to compare the number of visits to the learning-disability nurse made by the two groups of people and determine whether there is a statistically significant *difference* between the groups in their number of consultations.

You may remember that we got the output presented in Figure 10.1.

Group Statistics

	Sex of patient	N	Mean	Std. Deviation	Std. Error Mean
Number of consultations with learning disability nurse	Male	14	12.29	7.279	1.945
	Female	10	6.40	3.718	1.176

Independent Samples Test

		Levene's Test for Equality of Variances		t-test for Equality of Means						95% Confidence Interval of the Difference	
		F	Sig.	t	Df	Sig. (2-tailed)	Mean Difference	Std. Error Difference	Lower	Upper
Number of consultations with learning disability nurse	Equal variances assumed	2.428	.133	2.338	22	.029	5.886	2.517	.665	11.106
	Equal variances not assumed			2.589	20.315	.017	5.886	2.273	1.149	10.623

Figure 10.1 SPSS independent-samples t-test output: examining whether there is a statistically significant difference between males and females in their number of consultations among a sample of 24 individuals

We initially would have reported the following from this output:

An independent-samples *t*-test was used to examine statistically significant differences between males and females in terms of the number of consultations they had with the learning disability nurse. Males (mean = 12.29, S.D. = 7.3) scored statistically significantly higher ($t(22) = 2.34$, $p = 0.029$) than females (mean = 6.40, S.D. = 3.7) in terms of their number of consultations with the learning disability nurse. This finding suggests the males have statistically significantly more consultations with the learning disability nurse than do females.

However, an independent-samples *t*-test in SPSS also gives the confidence interval (as it does too in a paired-samples *t*-test). In SPSS this is given as a lower score and an upper score and the interval between these two numbers. Therefore you may find that researchers present these figures alongside their findings to give some indication of the confidence interval. Here the lower value is 0.665 and the upper value is 11.106. The confidence interval is worked out by subtracting the lower value from the upper value; here 11.106 − 0.665 = 10.441. Therefore the confidence interval is 10.441.

Now you may not think reporting this is particularly useful on its own. However, let us imagine that another study was carried out and looked at the same variables but this time in a sample that was ten times as large, with 240 people. Imagine we got the output shown in Figure 10.2.

As we can see from this output, without our confidence levels our write-up would be similar: the means for each group are identical, as is our conclusion, that there is a

Group Statistics

	Sex of patient	N	Mean	Std. Deviation	Std. Error Mean
Number of consultations with learning disability nurse	Male	140	12.29	7.040	.595
	Female	100	6.40	3.545	.354

Independent Samples Test

		Levene's Test for Equality of Variances		t-test for Equality of Means					95% Confidence Interval of the Difference	
		F	Sig.	t	Df	Sig. (2-tailed)	Mean Difference	Std. Error Difference	Lower	Upper
Number of consultations with learning disability nurse	Equal variances assumed	26.268	.000	7.690	238	.000	5.886	.765	4.378	7.393
	Equal variances not assumed			8.498	216.836	.000	5.886	.693	4.521	7.251

Figure 10.2 SPSS independent-samples *t*-test output: examining whether there is a statistically significant difference between males and females in their number of consultations among a sample of 240 individuals.

significant difference between males and females. Therefore confidence intervals would be useful to report here to help the reader. Here the upper value is 7.393 and the lower value is 4.378. Therefore the confidence interval is 3.015. This is lower than was found in the sample of 24 people and therefore indicates a greater level of confidence in the findings (in other words, a lower margin of error).

This brings us to the main point to remember about confidence intervals. Confidence intervals are said to be wide if they contain a large (or larger) range of values (for example, 0.665 to 11.106), and narrow if they contain a small (smaller) range of values (for example, 4.378 to 7.393). The wider the interval, the less confidence you have in the findings, as with the smaller sample.

● Things to do with confidence intervals

Before we end this chapter we are going to introduce to two things that you are likely to come across at some point in your career if you are going to carry out research. This is how to calculate confidence intervals from sample sizes, and how you can calculate required sample sizes from research from confidence intervals. Again, we are going to provide a simplified version of this for you, but it should give you confidence (no pun intended) when you first come across these things in the literature or in your career.

Calculating confidence intervals from sample sizes

First is finding your confidence interval. In Table 10.2, we gave you some broad estimates, but you can work out your confidence interval from sample sizes This is usually done using online calculators such as that at www.surveysystem.com/sscalc.htm (outlined in Figure 10.3). In this calculator the confidence level is set at 95 per cent and the percentage at 50 by default (Figure 10.3a). Unless you know otherwise, or need a higher confidence level, you can leave these as they are (you may learn more about these ideas in advanced statistics or research methods classes). As you can see from Figures 10.3(b) and (c), by changing the sample size (from 200 to 350, and then to 555), the confidence intervals decrease from 6.93 to 5.24 and then to 4.16.

Whenever you need to work out a confidence interval in future, you can simply go to this website to work it out.

Calculating sample sizes from confidence intervals

Calculating sample sizes from confidence intervals is considered a much more useful tool than vice versa, and if you are starting out in research you may find this idea useful. Look at Table 10.3. These are the confidence levels that accompany sample size at the 95 per cent probability level. You can see that if you collected a sample of 1,000 cases, your expected confidence interval would be 3 per cent. If you collected a sample of 2,000 cases, you have a confidence interval of 2 per cent. By doubling the sample

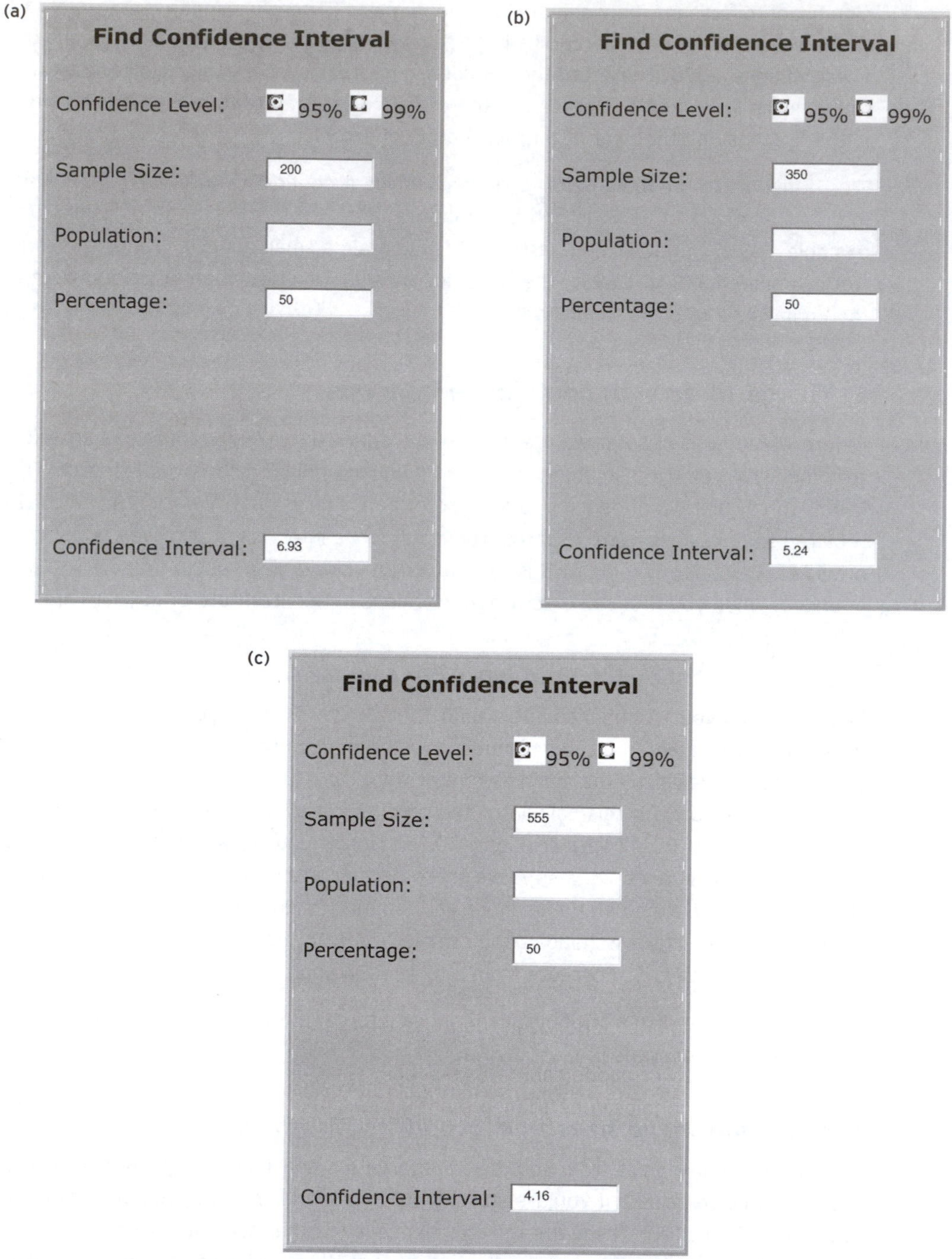

(a)

Find Confidence Interval

Confidence Level: ☑ 95% ☐ 99%

Sample Size: 200

Population:

Percentage: 50

Confidence Interval: 6.93

(b)

Find Confidence Interval

Confidence Level: ☑ 95% ☐ 99%

Sample Size: 350

Population:

Percentage: 50

Confidence Interval: 5.24

(c)

Find Confidence Interval

Confidence Level: ☑ 95% ☐ 99%

Sample Size: 555

Population:

Percentage: 50

Confidence Interval: 4.16

Figure 10.3 *Confidence interval calculator at www.surveysystem.com/sscalc.htm (Creative Research Systems, 2003)*

Table 10.3 Confidence intervals that accompany sample size at the 95 per cent probability level

Survey sample size	Confidence interval at the 95% probability level
2,000	2
1,000	3
800	3
600	4
400	5
200	7
100	10
50	14

to 2,000, the confidence interval only decreases from ±3 per cent to ±2 per cent. So you can imagine, as a researcher, we might ask the necessity of doubling our workload.

Consequently, many researchers like to determine before they start their research the sample size that will needed to establish a certain confidence interval. For example, opinion pollsters (such as MORI) will always tend to collect data from around 1,000–2,000 people because they always work within a margin of error of 2–3 per cent.

In the same way, we can do this in research using another online calculator at www.surveysystem.com/sscalc.htm, as outlined in Figure 10.4. Here, 95 per cent is a default setting, and all you need enter are your confidence interval and the size of the population you are dealing with. A population is all the people who fall within a particular category. Therefore all the people in a hospital are the population of that hospital. Or all the people with a particular illness (say, chronic obstructive pulmonary disease) represent the population of people with chronic obstructive pulmonary disease. A sample is a subset of a population. Therefore all the people in a particular ward are a sample of the population of a hospital. Or all the people who have chronic obstructive pulmonary disease in Koppers *et al.*'s study outlined earlier are a sample of people with chronic obstructive pulmonary disease.

Normally if you don't know the size of your population, that is, if you think you are sampling from a population of the general public in a particular area, then as a general rule you put 20,000 in the **Population:** box (because the sample size required doesn't change much for populations larger than 20,000). However, there are times when you might know the size of the general population, for example if you are sampling changes or opinions from a few wards in a hospital of 1,000 people. Again you would look for some guidance on this from your lecturers or your colleagues when deciding this. However, we've run through some examples to illustrate this.

Figures 10.4(a) and (b) show that the number of people you need varies with the confidence interval you require. So, for example, in Figure 10.4(a), if we wanted to examine significance findings at 95 per cent and wanted a confidence interval (margin of error)

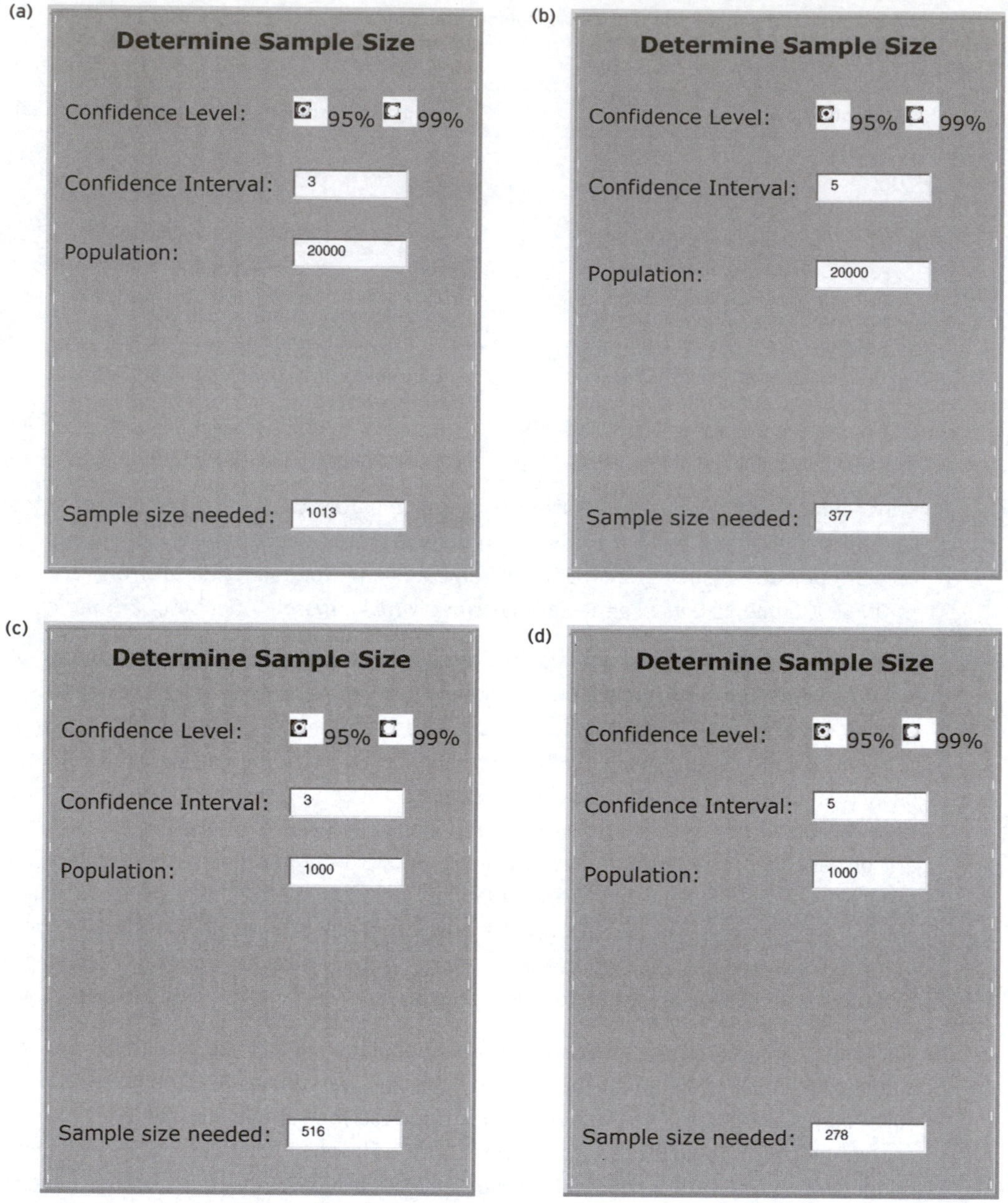

(a)
Determine Sample Size

Confidence Level: ⊙ 95% ☐ 99%

Confidence Interval: `3`

Population: `20000`

Sample size needed: `1013`

(b)
Determine Sample Size

Confidence Level: ⊙ 95% ☐ 99%

Confidence Interval: `5`

Population: `20000`

Sample size needed: `377`

(c)
Determine Sample Size

Confidence Level: ⊙ 95% ☐ 99%

Confidence Interval: `3`

Population: `1000`

Sample size needed: `516`

(d)
Determine Sample Size

Confidence Level: ⊙ 95% ☐ 99%

Confidence Interval: `5`

Population: `1000`

Sample size needed: `278`

Figure 10.4 *Sample size calculator at www.surveysystem.com/sscalc.htm (Creative Research Systems, 2003)*

from our results of 3 per cent, we would need to question 1,013 people. If, however, as in Figure 10.4(b), we wanted a confidence interval of 5 per cent, we would only need to survey 377 people.

In Figure 10.4(c) we have changed the population value to 1,000. Let us say, for example, we are sampling people with a particular illness. Therefore if we wanted to examine significance findings at 95 per cent and wanted a confidence interval (margin of error) from our results of 3 per cent, we would need to sample 516 people with the illness. Figure 10.4(d) shows that, if among the same population we wanted a confidence interval (margin of error) from our results of 5 per cent, we would need to sample 278 people with the illness.

There are many online confidence interval and sample size calculators,[1] but links to webpages can change. Therefore if the links we have given so far are broken, type 'calculating confidence interval' or 'calculating margin of error' into an internet search engine and you will come across an internet resource that does this.

Summary

In this chapter we have covered:

✔ **statistical and clinical significance, and how these relate to effect size and percentage improvement;**

✔ **hypothesis testing and confidence intervals, and how these two concepts are used in the literature to provide context (frameworks) to statistical findings.**

It is important to remember that we haven't gone into great detail on these subjects, as sometimes they are associated with advanced statistical thinking or research methods. However, as these commonly reported alongside statistics in the nursing literature we thought we would give you an overview of them. You will see when you look at the literature that people don't always consider ideas around statistical and clinical significance, hypothesis testing and confidence intervals; however, when they do, you will be aware of what these things mean.

---

[1] For example, Raosoft's sample size calculator is provided at www.raosoft.com/samplesize.html.

Appendix: Summary

With that we bring the book to a close. But before we close entirely, let us just check your progression in statistics. On each of the sections in the checklist below, rate yourself from 0 to 10 (0 being not very good at all, 5 average and 10 perfect) on your knowledge of the areas covered in each chapter.

LEARNING CHECKLIST

Score

Chapter 2 Variables

This chapter teaches you some core ideas that underlie statistics. From completing this chapter you should be able to:

- Outline what variables are and how they are evident in many aspects of investigation
- Describe how variables are viewed by investigators
- Demonstrate the form variables take in SPSS for Windows by way of creating a datafile
- Use SPSS for Windows to create and save a datafile of variables   ___/10

Chapter 3 Descriptive statistics

This chapter teaches you ways of describing data. From completing this chapter you should be able to:

- Show a knowledge of frequency counts, averages, a measure of dispersion, bar charts and histograms, and how to obtain these statistics on SPSS for Windows
- Perform, in SPSS for Windows, techniques in statistics that allow you to alter the structure of your data: the Recode and Compute statements   ___/10

Chapter 4 Effective data cleaning and management

This chapter teaches you ways of managing statistical data. From completing this chapter you should be able to:

- Explain the concept of validity and why it is important in nursing research
- Demonstrate how research can be made less valid by not adhering to principles of effective data management and cleaning
- Use descriptive statistics to look for errors in data entry or coding   ___/10

Chapter 5 Critical appraisal of analysis and reporting of descriptive statistics

This chapter teaches you ways of thinking further about descriptive statistics. From completing this chapter you should be able to:

- Explain the importance of critical appraisal as a process for evaluating the strengths and limitations of a study

- Outline a critical appraisal framework for evaluating the use of descriptive statistics in a study
- Apply your critical appraisal skills by using the critical appraisal framework to evaluate a case study article   ___/10

Chapter 6 An introduction to inferential statistics

This chapter introduces you to a series of statistical tests called inferential statistics. From completing this chapter you should be able to:

- Outline what is meant by terms such as distribution, probability and statistical significance testing
- Outline the importance of probability values in determining statistical significance
- Outline the decision-making process about what informs the use of parametric and non-parametric statistical tests
- Determine a statistically significant result
- Carry out the chi-square statistical test using SPSS for Windows   ___/10

Chapter 7 Correlational statistics

This chapter teaches you about two types of inferential statistical tests known as correlation statistics. From completing this chapter you should be able to demonstrate the rationale for, the procedure for and the interpretation in SPSS of Windows of two inferential statistical tests:

- Pearson product–moment correlation coefficient
- Spearman's rho correlation   ___/10

Chapter 8 Comparing average scores: statistics for all sorts of groups and occasions

This chapter teaches you about four types of inferential statistical test that are concerned with examining differences. From completing this chapter you should be able to demonstrate the rationale for the procedure for and the interpretation in SPSS for Windows of the following four inferential statistical tests:

- Independent-samples t-test
- Paired-samples t-test
- Wilcoxon sign-ranks test
- Mann–Whitney U test   ___/10

Chapter 9 Critical appraisal of analysis and reporting of inferential statistics

This chapter helps you understand the use of inferential statistics in research. It addresses the use of inferential statistics in nursing research papers and the nursing literature. The chapter contains sections which ask you to interpret examples from the literature. From completing this chapter you should be able to:

- Use critical appraisal to evaluate the reporting of inferential statistics
- Apply a critical appraisal framework to evaluate research and research articles   ___/10

Chapter 10 Advanced thinking with probability and statistics

This chapter teaches you about thinking further around inferential statistical tests. From completing this chapter you should be able to demonstrate knowledge of:

- Statistical and clinical significance, and how these relate to effect size and percentage improvement
- Hypothesis testing and confidence intervals, and how these two concepts are used in the literature to provide context to statistical findings   ___/10

Where you have rated yourself below 5 we suggest that you revisit that chapter soon and cover the material again. You can also reuse this checklist and scoring system every now and then as an ongoing guide to the areas of statistics where your knowledge requires a little brushing up.

Glossary

Alternative hypothesis A hypothesis that refers to a statement that the results found in a study are expected to show a statistically significant relationship.

Bar chart A chart used to summarise categorical-type data in graphical form.

Categorical data Data comprising categories that have no numerical value or order.

Categorical-type data A term used in this book to describe data that have been put into categories and that do not have any numerical properties.

Chi-square The chi-square test of association allows the comparison of two categorical-type data to determine whether there is any relationship between them.

Clinical significance A measure of whether a study finding actually matters in the real world.

Confidence interval A confidence interval gives an estimated range of values from which the confidence range of the findings can be considered.

Confounding variable A variable that is linked to a participant's characteristics (for example, the extent to which a participant may believe in a certain treatment).

Continuous data A set of data is said to be continuous if the values or observations belonging to it may take on any value. Continuous data, unlike discrete data, can have decimal points.

Continuous-type data A term used in this book to describe data that have been ordered numerically or given numerical properties in some way.

Control group A group that does not receive the intervention that is to be tested in a research study; the group is used as a comparator for the experimental group.

Dependent groups/samples Samples that are related in some way. For example, they may be the same individuals 'before' and 'after' an experimental intervention, or different individuals may be matched across groups (for example, similar sex, age or ethnicity).

Dependent variable A variable that the researcher believes might be influenced or modified by some treatment or intervention.

Descriptive statistics Statistics that are techniques used to summarise and describe data.

Discrete data Continuous-type data. A set of data is said to be discrete if the data values are distinct and separate and represent whole numbers. Discrete data, unlike continuous data, cannot have decimal points.

Ecological validity The extent to which findings can be generalised beyond the current situation.

Effect size The term given to a group of indices that measure the magnitude of a statistical finding.

Expected frequencies In a contingency table (Crosstabs in SPSS), the expected frequencies are the frequencies that would be expected to be obtained in each cell of the table from the sample if everything was random. Expected frequencies are spread evenly across the cells. Most commonly used with a chi-square test.

Experimental group A group that receives an intervention that is to be tested in the research study.

External validity If a study has external validity, its results will generalise to the larger population.

Extraneous variable A variable outside of the participants' sphere of influence (for example, noise/heat in a room), which can bias how participants react in a study.

Frequency table A way of summarising data by assigning a number of occurrences to each level of variable.

Histogram A graphical display of frequencies of scores used commonly with continuous-type data.

Hypothesis Suggested explanation or statements of the possible relationship between variables. (Plural: hypotheses.)

Independent groups/samples Those samples selected from the same population or different populations but which are considered independent of (unrelated to) each other (for example, men and women).

Independent-samples _t_-test A statistical test used to evaluate the differences in means between two to independent groups (also called independent-groups _t_-test).

Independent variable A variable which is measured or selected by the researcher to examine influence on another variable (dependent variable).

Inferential statistics Comprises the use of statistical tests to make inferences, or generalise, concerning the nature of the relationship between variables.

Internal validity A study has internal validity if it properly demonstrates the relationship between variables.

Interquartile range (IQR) A measure of the range of scores between the upper and the lower quartiles.

Interval data/variables Have levels that are ordered and numerical. Interval data are distinct from ratio data as interval data have no absolute zero (that is, absence of what is being measured).

Intransitive response A logically inconsistent response. Such data should be discarded with caution though, as people do behave illogically inconsistent ways and such responses are still possible.

Mann–Whitney _U_ test A non-parametric statistical test for comparing scores of two groups on a continuous-type variable.

Mean An average statistic worked out by adding all the values together, and then dividing this total by the number of values (for example, the mean of 6 and 4 would be 10 divided by 2, which is 5).

Median The value that appears halfway in a set of data when those data have been ordered by value (for example, in the set of values 1, 2, 3, 4, 5, the median is 3).

Mode The most frequently occurring value in data (for example, in the set of values 1, 2, 2, 2, 5, the mode is 2).

Negatively skewed distribution A distribution of scores in which the majority of scores fall to the right of the distribution.

Nominal variable A variable whose levels are distinct from one another.

Non-parametric statistical tests Non-parametric tests are often used instead of parametric counterparts when certain assumptions about the underlying population are questionable, for example when continuous-type data are not normally distributed.

Normal distribution A distribution of scores shaped liked a bell curve in which the same number or percentage of scores fall on either side of the centre of the distribution.

Null hypothesis A hypothesis that refers to a statement that the results found in a study are no different from what might have occurred as a result of chance.

Observed frequencies In a contingency table (Crosstabs in SPSS), the observed frequencies are the frequencies actually obtained in each cell of the table, from the sample. Most commonly used with a chi-square test.

Ordinal data/variables Data whose values/observations can be ranked (put in order) or have a rating scale attached.

Paired-samples _t_-test A parametric statistical test to determine whether there is a significant difference between the average values of the same variable made under two different conditions among the same sample. Also known as a dependent-groups _t_-test.

Paired/matched samples Two samples in which the members are clearly paired or matched.

Parametric statistical test A statistical test that requires that the normality assumptions are met, for example that continuous data form a normal distribution.

Pearson correlation coefficient A correlation coefficient (r) is a number between −1 and +1 which indicates the degree to which two variables are statistically significantly related.

Percentiles Values that divide a sample of data into 100 groups (i.e. 100 per cent), each representing 1 per cent.

Pie chart A way of summarising a set of categorical-type data.

Population Any entire collection of people.

Population validity The extent to which the findings can be generalised to other populations of people.

Positively skewed distribution A distribution of scores in which the majority of scores fall to the left of the distribution.

Probability value The probability value (p-value) in a statistical hypothesis test is the probability of getting a value of the test statistic higher than that observed by chance alone.

Quartiles Values that divide a sample of data into four groups containing equal numbers of observations.

Random sample Data that have been drawn from a population in such a way that each piece of data had an equal opportunity to appear in the sample.

Range The numerical distance between two numbers. For example, the range between 1 and 5 is 4.

Ratio data/variables Have levels that are ordered and numerical. Ratio data are numerical but are distinct from interval data as ratio data have an absolute zero (that is, absence of what is being measured).

Sample A group of units or cases (for example, people, test results) selected from a larger group (the population) of units/cases. Researchers study samples in the hope of being able to draw conclusions about the larger group.

Sampling error The error caused by the selection of a sample.

Semi-interquartile range (SIQR) A measure of the range of scores between the upper and the lower quartiles divided by 2. Also a measure of the extent to which a set of scores vary. Often accompanies the reporting of the median.

Spearman correlation coefficient A correlation coefficient (*rho* or *r*) between −1 and +1 which indicates the degree to which two variables are related.

Standard deviation A measure of the extent to which a set of scores vary. Often accompanies the reporting of the mean.

Statistical inference Statistical inference makes use of information from a sample to draw conclusions (inferences) about the population from which the sample was taken.

Statistical significance A result is statistically significant if it is probable that it has not occurred by chance.

Type I error When the use of a statistical test incorrectly reports that it has found a statistically significant result where none really exists.

Type II error When the use of a statistical test incorrectly reports that it has not found a statistically significant result where one really exists.

Variability The extent to which scores within a particular sample vary. It is described using the range, the semi-interquartile range and the standard deviation.

Wilcoxon sign-ranks test A non-parametric statistical test for comparing scores on the same continuous-type variable on two occasions (or for comparing matched groups).

References

Astor, R. (2001) 'Detecting pain in people with profound learning disabilities', *Nursing Times* 97(40): 38-9.

Barr, W. (2000) 'Characteristics of severely mentally ill patients in and out of contact with community mental health services', *Journal of Advanced Nursing*, 31: 1189-1198.

Beck, A.T., Steer, R.A. and Garbin, M.G. (1988) 'Psychometric properties of the Beck Depression Inventory: twenty-five years of evaluation', *Clinical Psychology Review*, 8: 77-100.

Bernal, C. (2005) 'Maintenance of oral health in people with learning disabilities', *Nursing Times*, 101(6): 40-42.

Booth-Kewley, S. and Friedman, H.S. (1987) 'Psychological predictors of heart disease: a quantitative review', *Psychological Bulletin*, 101: 343-362.

Boynton, P. (2005) *The Research Companion: A Practical Guide to the Social and Health Sciences.* Hove: Psychology Press/Brunner-Routledge.

British Heart Foundation (2004) *Coronary Heart Disease Statistics*. London: BHF.

Brown, S.A., Harrist, R.B., Villagomez, E.T., Segura, M., Barton, S.A. and Hanis, C.L. (2000) 'Gender and treatment differences in knowledge, health beliefs, and metabolic control in Mexican Americans with type B diabetes', *Diabetes Educator*, 26: 425-428.

Bush, T. (2005) 'Reviewing case management in community psychiatric care', *Nursing Times*, 101(38): 40-43.

Clegg, F. (1982) *Simple Statistics: A Coursebook for the Social Sciences*. Cambridge: Cambridge University Press.

Cohen, J. (1988) *Statistical Power Analysis for the Behavioral Sciences*, 2nd edn. Hillsdale, NJ: Lawrence Erlbaum Associates.

Cox, J.L., Holden, J.M. and Sagovsky, R. (1987) 'Detection of postnatal depression: development of the 10-item Edinburgh Postnatal Depression Scale', *British Journal of Psychiatry*, 150: 782-876.

Creative Research Systems (2003) The Survey System. Available at www.surveysystem.com/sscalc.htm. Accessed May 2006.

Diamantopoulos, A. and Schlegelmilch, B.B. (2000) *Taking the Fear Out of Data Analysis*. London: Thomson Learning.

Diggle, L. (2005) 'Understanding and dealing with parental vaccine concerns', *Nursing Times*, 101(46): 26-28.

Dunbar, H. (2001) 'Improving the management of asthma in under-fives', *Nursing Times*, 97(31): 36.

Earnhart, B. (2003) Data training. University of Iowa, Dept of Sociology. Available at www.uiowa.edu/~soc/datarespect/data_training_frm.html.Accessed October 2006.

Finlay, I.G., Maughan, T.S. and Webster, D.J. (1998) 'A randomized controlled study of portfolio learning in undergraduate cancer education', *Medical Education*, 32: 172-176.

Forde, F., Frame, M., Hanlon, P., Machean, G., Nolan, D. *et al.* (2005) 'Optimum number of sessions for depression and anxiety', *Nursing Times*, 101(43): 36-40.

Gibbs, G. (1988) *Learning by Doing*. Sheffield: Further Education Unit.

Goodman, L. and Keeton, E. (2005) 'Choice in the diet of people with learning difficulties', *Nursing Times*, 101(14): 28-29.

Hainsworth, T. (2004) 'The role of exercise in falls prevention for older patients', *Nursing Times*, 100(18): 28-29.

Hanley, J. (2006) 'The assessment and treatment of postnatal depression', *Nursing Times*, 102(1): 24-26.

Hobgood. C., Villani, J. and Quattlebaum, R. (2005) 'Impact of emergency department volume on registered nurse time at the bedside', *Annals of Emergency Medicine*, 46: 481-489.

Hodgkins, C., Rose, D. and Rose, J. (2005) 'A collaborative approach to reducing stress among staff', *Nursing Times*, 101(28): 35-37.

Jackson, G.A. (2002) 'Behaviour problems and assessment in dementia', *Nursing Times*, 98(47): 32.

Koppers, R.J.H., Vos, P.J.E., Boot, C.R.L. and Folgering, H.T.M. (2006) 'Exercise performance improves in patients with COPD due to respiratory muscle endurance training', *Chest*, 129: 886-892.

Loharuka, S. (2005) 'Incontinence and falls in older people: is there a link?', *Nursing Times*, 101(47): 52.

Marshall, K., Nelson, S. and Sykes, C. (2005) 'Analysing and improving a rapid-access chest pain clinic', *Nursing Times*, 101(41): 32-33.

McEwen, A., Cooper, S. and Clayworth, S. (2005) 'Are ward sisters and charge nurses able to fulfil their role?', *Nursing Times*, 101(29): 38-41.

Mykletun, A., Stordal, E. and Dahl, AA. (2001) 'Hospital Anxiety and Depression (HAD) scale: factor structure, item analyses and internal consistency in a large population', *British Journal of Psychiatry*, 179: 540-544.

Naerde, A., Tambs, K., Mathiesen, K.S., Dalgard, O.S. and Samuelsen, S.O. (2000) 'Symptoms of anxiety and depression among mothers of pre-school children: effect of chronic strain related to children and child care-taking', *Journal of Affective Disorders*, 58: 181-199.

Nairn, S., O'Brien, E., Traynor, V., Williams, G., Chapple, M. and Johnson, S. (2006) 'Student nurses' knowledge, skills and attitudes towards the use of portfolios in a school of nursing', *Journal of Clinical Nursing*. In press.

Nursing Times (2005) 'Insomnia', 101(39): 25.

Perdue, C. (2003) 'Falls in older people: taking a multidisciplinary approach', *Nursing Times*, 99(31): 28-30.

Polit, D.F. and Hungler, B.P. (1997) *Essential of Nursing Research: Methods, Appraisals, and Ultilization*, 4th edn. Philadelphia, PA: Lippincott-Raven.

Polit, D.F. and Hungler, B.P. (1999) *Nursing Research: Principles and Methods*. Philadelphia, PA: Lippincott Williams & Wilkins.

Population Reference Bureau (2004) *World Population Data Sheet*. Washington, DC: PRB.

Powell, H., Murray, G. and McKenzie, K. (2004) 'Staff perceptions of community learning disability nurses' role', *Nursing Times*, 100(19): 40-42.

Rosenthal, R. (1991) *Meta-analytic Procedures for Social Research*, rev. edn. Newbury Park, CA: Sage.

Rugg, K. (2004) 'Childhood obesity: its incidence, consequences and prevention', *Nursing Times*, 100(3): 28.

Smith, M. (2005) 'Does encouragement boost visual acuity testing results?', *Nursing Times*, 101(38): 38-41.

Spence, W. and El-Ansari, W. (2004) 'Portfolio assessment: practice teachers' early experience', *Nurse Education Today*, 24: 388-401.

Ware, J.E., Kosinski, M. and Keller, S.D. (1994) *SF-36 Physical and Mental Component Summary Measures: A User's Manual*. Boston, MA: New England Medical Center, The Health Institute.

Ware, J.E., Kosinski, M. and Dewey, J.E. (2000) *How to Score Version Two of the SF-36 Health Survey*. Lincoln, RI: QualityMetric, Inc.

Williams, G.A. and Laungani, P. (1999) 'Analysis of teamwork in an NHS community trust: an empirical study', *Journal of InterProfessional Care*, 13: 19-28.

Wright, D.B. and Williams, S. (2003) 'How to produce a bad results section', *Psychologist*, 16(12): 646-648.

Index